The Right Therapy for Neurological Disorders

Frontiers of Neurology and Neuroscience

Vol. 39

Series Editor

J. Bogousslavsky   Montreux

The Right Therapy for Neurological Disorders

From Randomized Trials to Clinical Practice

Volume Editors

E. Beghi Milan

G. Logroscino Bari/Tricase

18 figures, 1 in color, and 16 tables, 2016

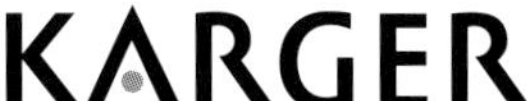

Basel · Freiburg · Paris · London · New York · Chennai · New Delhi ·
Bangkok · Beijing · Shanghai · Tokyo · Kuala Lumpur · Singapore · Sydney

Frontiers of Neurology and Neuroscience

Vols. 1–18 were published as Monographs in Clinical Neuroscience

Ettore Beghi, MD
Laboratory of Neurological Disorders
ICRRS – Mario Negri Institute for Pharmacological
Research
IT–20156 Milan (Itlay)

Giancarlo Logroscino, MD
Unit of Neurodegenerative Diseases
Department of Clinical Research in Neurology
University of Bari 'Aldo Moro'
'Pia, Fondazione Cardinale G. Panico'
IT–73039 Tricase (Italy)

Library of Congress Cataloging-in-Publication Data

Names: Beghi, E. (Ettore), editor. | Logroscino, G. (Giancarlo), editor.
Title: The right therapy for neurological disorders : from randomized trials
    to clinical practice / volume editors, E. Beghi, G. Logroscino.
Other titles: Frontiers of neurology and neuroscience ; v. 39. 1660-4431
Description: Basel ; New York : Karger, 2016. | Series: Frontiers of
    neurology and neuroscience, ISSN 1660-4431 ; vol. 39 | Includes
    bibliographical references and indexes.
Identifiers: LCCN 2016019282| ISBN 9783318058642 (hard cover : alk. paper) |
    ISBN 9783318058659 (e-ISBN)
Subjects: | MESH: Nervous System Diseases--drug therapy | Randomized
    Controlled Trials as Topic | Drug Evaluation--methods | Treatment Outcome
    | Evidence-Based Medicine--methods
Classification: LCC RM315 | NLM WL 140 | DDC 616.8/0461--dc23 LC record available at
https://lccn.loc.gov/2016019282

Bibliographic Indices. This publication is listed in bibliographic services, including Current Contents® and Index Medicus.

© Copyright 2016 by S. Karger AG, P.O. Box, CH-4009 Basel (Switzerland)
www.karger.com
Printed on acid-free and non-aging paper (ISO 9706)
ISSN 1660–4431
e-ISSN 1662–2804
ISBN 978–3–318–05864–2
e-ISBN 978–3–318–05865–9

Contents

Foreword

The right therapy needs to be evidence based for neurological disorders just like all the diseases that afflict humankind. Evidence-based medicine requires randomized clinical trials (RCTs) to establish the efficacy and effectiveness of therapeutic interventions. RCTs, today mostly focused on drug evaluation, need to be extended to other treatments too, such as medical devices, electrical stimulation, surgery, nutrition, and rehabilitation practices. Moreover, many current therapeutic practices are still largely based on tradition and impressions, not on evidence. Even when a treatment is based on RCTs, frequently too few patients are enrolled and there may be biases that undermine the significance of the results.

This all reflects the vast economic interests that today surround medicine as a whole, and obviously also neurology. RCTs need to be conducted by independent organizations that may offer advantages over trials run by industry.

It may be worth very briefly mentioning the principal bias that is frequently detected. Selection of the population is certainly one of the main problems because it is very hard to balance the need for a homogeneous group of patients while at the same time covering patients likely to be encountered in current clinical practice. This usually results in an important imbalance concerning age and sex. Today almost 70% of drugs are used by patients older than 65; however, this population is underrepresented in most RCTs. These patients are no longer likely to have only a single disease, but because of their age they present polymorbidity and require polytherapy. These conditions are far removed from the clear situation of the RCT usually carried out in middle-aged males.

Females are also underrepresented in clinical trials and even when they are present it is difficult to find out from the trial publications whether they were even affected by the intervention similarly or differently from males.

The abuse of placebo is also very frequent in contrast with the ethical Declaration of Helsinki which requires comparisons with the best available treatment to avoid patients risking undue progression of their disease. Unfortunately, the approval of new drugs does not require comparative studies. In fact, the European directive specifies three requirements: quality, efficacy, and safety, but it does not require 'added therapeutic value'. If it did, drugs would be better selected. A consequence of the fact that the European directive does not require superiority is that RCTs often set out to prove only 'noninferiority', which is ethically unacceptable because the null hypothesis is that the tested drug or treatment is worse than the treatment already available. Usually, it is promised that the noninferior efficacy is compensated by other advantages such as less toxicity. However, RCTs are mainly designed to establish benefits while adverse reactions can be detected only in clinical practice once the treatment has been available for several years.

Clinical interventions must offer an outcome that is beneficial for patients, but RCTs often employ surrogate end points which are not always relevant to the patients' quality of life. A typical case is a drug that reduces the volume of a tumor but does not affect what is important for the patient, i.e. overall survival.

Since RCTs will never be perfect, it is very important for the protocol to be registered in an easily accessible site and that the results always get published and raw data made available, under certain conditions, to independent investigators.

One of the main difficulties is making sure that results are not only dealt with in the scientific literature, but that they can be translated into clinical practice. It would therefore be useful if publications could include brief summaries of the clinical significance of the results. In particular, clinicians may appreciate knowing clearly how many patients need to be treated to ensure a therapeutic benefit in one patient.

This book, coordinated by Beghi and Logroscino, is a sort of compendium relating most of the principles of reliable RCTs to specific neurological diseases. The articles, written by specialized neurologists, have the merit of touching on important aspects of RCTs with a clear, critical approach. Neurologists involved in clinical trials will certainly learn a lot from this book, which should become a basic text for all neurological courses dealing with evidence-based neurology.

Silvio Garattini, Milan

Preface

The Treatment of the Neurological Disorders

Neurological disorders represent a relevant and ever-increasing fraction of the global burden of disease [1, 2]. As most neurological disorders are chronic and aging-related, with the increase of life expectancy and a decrease in age-specific mortality we expect a significant increase of their incidence and prevalence in the decades to come. The increase in frequency of neurodegenerative disorders will be a major part of another important phenomenon: the increase of life lived with disabilities. The trend will determine an increasing load on medical and social systems both in low- and high-income countries. There is thus a desperate need for successful preventive and therapeutic (curative) measures. During the last decades, a number of effective drugs have been made available to the benefit of patients with several neurological disorders, such as epilepsy, Parkinson's disease, and multiple sclerosis. However, these drugs are symptomatic and at present there are no compounds apparently capable to abate or at least slow the progression of these diseases.

The lack of effective therapies has determined an increased role of prevention trials, especially in neurodegenerative disorders like Alzheimer's disease. In the past decades, as with cardio- and cerebrovascular diseases, interventions modifying lifestyle (primarily physical activity and diet) have been explored for the prevention of cognitive decline in randomized clinical trials of individuals mostly in their midlife years. More recently, pharmacological prevention trials have also been started.

The picture is made even more complicated by the use of diagnostic tests with increasing levels of sophistication, which have brought the anticipation of diagnosis for some diseases to a subclinical (preclinical) level. In addition, genetic tests have added to the complexity of the spectrum of each disease with results not always understandable, given the frequent inconsistency of the genotype-phenotype correlations. Genetic tests have been rarely used in the stratification process in randomized clinical trials, with the sole exception of apolipoprotein E (APOE) in Alzheimer's disease trials [3]. The spectrum of disease phenotypes has been largely expanded in the last few years due to new insights from genetics. A good example is the C9orf72 gene discovery that has linked frontotemporal dementia and amyotrophic lateral sclerosis [4].

In addition, epidemiological studies done in well-defined cohorts of patients with neurodegenerative disorders with prolonged follow-up have given further impulse to the characterization of the heterogeneity of chronic neurological disorders. All this is challenged by the external validity of the results of traditional clinical trials that are obtained from strictly homogeneous samples and, as such, are not applicable to all the aspects of the disease spectrum. The consequence is that the same treatment is offered to patients in whom the disease has significantly different levels of severity (including cases that might never become symptomatic).

This is further complicated by the need to combine the clinical impact of the study results with the patients' values and the interests of the pharmaceutical companies. Frequently, the needs expressed by the patients do not coincide with the expectations of the caring physicians, while big pharma prefers to invest in fields where the profit is not negligible. This reflects, on one side, the tendency to refrain from developing compounds to be used in rare diseases and, on the other side, to prefer the development of 'me-too' drugs or to magnify small, sometimes only subclinical, effects in the attempt to justify the earliest possible treatment.

Upon this background, a discussion has been started on the structure of the randomized trial to verify if and to what extent the present designs are suitable for proving the efficacy of an experimental treatment. Neurological conditions have peculiar features that may require the use of adaptive designs to address (and adjust for) the heterogeneous phenotypes and the differing levels of disease severity.

In view of the increasing number of biomarkers, disease-specific study end points must be defined, paying attention to the clinical relevance of each biological parameter. Then, in addition to the caring physicians' therapeutic expectations, patients' and caregivers' needs must be more deeply considered when assessing treatment efficacy.

These aspects are the main objects of this book, the intent of which is to outline all the problems posed by acute and chronic neurological conditions and offer discussion points to the scientific community for the improvement of preventive and therapeutic strategies. International leaders in the field of neurological disorders have been invited to highlight this complex issue with the intent to provide a background for identifying the right therapy for neurological disorders in the near future. These experts have accomplished their task with examples from their specific fields of expertise. However, far from driving the reader's attention away from the main focus of this book, these contributions help to shed light on the diverse and multifaceted aspects of major neurological diseases and provide scientists in charge of the design of therapeutic trials with all the elements needed to plan and conduct trials that can fulfill the unmet needs of scientists, caring physicians, and patients.

Ettore Beghi, Milan
Giancarlo Logroscino, Bari/Tricase

References

1 Prince MJ, Wu F, Guo Y, et al: The burden of disease in older people and implications for health policy and practice. Lancet 2015;385:549–562.

2 Stovner LJ, Hoff JM, Svalheim S, Gilhus NE: Neurological disorders in the Global Burden of Disease 2010 study. Acta Neurol Scand Suppl 2014, pp 1–6.

3 Carrillo MC, Brashear HR, Logovinsky V, et al: Can we prevent Alzheimer's disease? Secondary 'prevention' trials in Alzheimer's disease. Alzheimers Dement 2013;9:123–131.

4 Wood H: A hexanucleotide repeat expansion in C9ORF72 links amyotrophic lateral sclerosis and frontotemporal dementia. Nat Rev Neurol 2011;7:595.

Beghi E, Logroscino G (eds): The Right Therapy for Neurological Disorders. From Randomized Trials to Clinical Practice.
Front Neurol Neurosci. Basel, Karger, 2016, vol 39, pp 1–7 (DOI: 10.1159/000445408)

The Basic Structure of a Randomized Clinical Trial

Ettore Beghi

Laboratory of Neurological Disorders, IRCCS-Mario Negri Institute for Pharmacological Research, Milan, Italy

Abstract

Background: According to the Directive 2001/20/EC of the European Union, a clinical trial is any investigation in human subjects intended to (1) discover or verify the clinical, pharmacological, and/or other pharmacodynamic effects of one or more investigational medicinal product(s), (2) identify any adverse reactions to one or more investigational medicinal product(s), (3) and/or study absorption, distribution, metabolism and excretion of one or more investigational medicinal product(s) with the object of ascertaining its (their) safety and/or efficacy. **Summary:** The major steps in the planning and conduction of a randomized clinical trial (RCT) include the definition of the study population, the random assignment of treatments, the choice of the measures of treatment effects, the duration of the experiment, the assessment of the tolerability and safety of the treatment, and the choice of alternative design models. In doing this, a constant reference will be made to the peculiarities (and diversities) of neurological disorders. **Key Messages:** An RCT is the best model to test the efficacy, tolerability, and safety of a drug, and reflects the need to disentangle the effects of the treatment from the effects of other prognostic variables. This requires a number of restrictions that are, at the same time, limitations for the application of the study results to the individuals who will receive the treatment in clinical practice.
© 2016 S. Karger AG, Basel

A randomized clinical trial (RCT) represents the best (and at present the only) model to assess the efficacy, tolerability, and safety of any treatment for all clinical conditions, including neurological disorders. The structure of the trial is based on the need to disentangle the effects of an experimental treatment (to be compared to one or more control treatments) from variables with prognostic significance, which may act as confounders. To perform this task, a number of restrictions must be considered in order to make the experimental and control groups highly comparable and to show statistically significant differences between the experimental groups and the controls in a relatively limited time frame. These strengths are, at the same time, limitations of RCTs and can be amended only in part, as indicated below.

The major steps in the planning and conduction of an RCT include the definition of the study population, the random assignment of treatments, the choice of the measures of treatment effects, the duration of the experiment, the assessment of the tolerability and safety of the treatment, and the choice of alternative design models. In doing this, a constant reference will be made to the peculiarities (and diversities) of neurological disorders. Other aspects of the RCT protocol will not be covered because the focus of this chapter is the scientific basis of the experimental procedure. These additional aspects include administration, funding, quality control, and infrastructure. Other sources can be addressed by those interested in regulatory matters (see www. ema.europa.eu).

Study Population

The choice of the study population represents a critical issue when assessing the effects of a treatment. In fact, when dealing with chronic diseases (as the majority of neurological disorders are), a marked heterogeneity in the severity and clinical characteristics of a disease is expected. Differences in the phenotype of the affected individuals may thus affect the outcome of the disease. For example, even in a severe clinical condition like amyotrophic lateral sclerosis (ALS), survival (a measure of treatment efficacy in this disease) may vary significantly across patients. Longer survival can be predicted by younger age, male sex, spinal onset, and suspected/possible ALS [1]. Different prognostic patterns are usually observed in patients with other chronic neurological disorders [2, 3] and require proper management to assess the net effect of treatment. The ideal approach should be to increase the sample size. However, this approach may be expensive, more difficult to organize, and time-consuming. The commonest way to overcome the heterogeneity of the study population consists of the exclusion of patients in whom disease severity and outcome differ from those of the majority of the affected individuals. These restrictions tend to remove part of the population, which is the object of the treatment, to isolate a fairly homogeneous sample which may not represent the entire origin population. An acceptable compromise is the stratification of the patients in separate subgroups in which the severity and outcome of the disease are fairly similar. For example, patients with ALS can be stratified by origin of symptoms (spinal vs. bulbar), an aspect of the disease found to impact outcome to a significant extent.

Another major issue with the study population is the selection of incident or prevalent cases. In most RCTs, patients represent samples of prevalent populations. In a prevalent population, newly diagnosed patients and patients with severe disease varieties tend to be underrepresented. Newly diagnosed patients are less likely to participate in clinical trials (except for studies dealing with drugs used for treatment start, like in epilepsy) and patients with severe disease are more likely to die before being included in the study. This is particularly true for life-threatening diseases like ALS or Huntington chorea. In this regard, patients included in RCTs may be mostly represented by individuals with long-lasting, slowly progressing disease. For these reasons, the recruitment of newly diagnosed (or incident) patients may be preferable. However, the intrinsic severity of the disease may vary across newly diagnosed patients and, as such, affect the outcome and the response to treatment, introducing a relevant source of bias in the event of an unbalanced distribution of patients according to disease severity. To overcome this potential bias, patients could be stratified according to known predefined prognostic markers. In patients with multiple sclerosis, the site of onset of symptoms may predict the course of the disease in terms of relapse and progression of functional disability [4]. Likewise, compared to generalized myasthenia, ocular myasthenia may have a more favorable prognosis

[5]. Patients should then be stratified according to the site of onset of symptoms provided that site has robust prognostic significance. By the same token, children, adults, and the elderly as well as patients with and without comorbidities should be randomized separately.

Diagnosis

A correct diagnosis is a prerequisite for the inclusion of a patient in an RCT. Although this concept may be intuitive, in clinical practice (and for most neurological disorders) the diagnosis is strongly dependent on clinical judgment. With the exception of infectious disorders and clinical conditions, like stroke, epilepsy, and multiple sclerosis, in which imaging studies are relevant diagnostic markers, the diagnosis rests upon subjective assessment and, as such, has limited validity and reliability. In an RCT, the inclusion of patients without a given disease or with differing disease varieties tends to dilute treatment effects and increase the placebo response. In patients with newly diagnosed epilepsy, one of the most plausible explanations of the lack of differences between carbamazepine and valproate given as monotherapy was that several patients with generalized seizures were misdiagnosed as having focal seizures (the target of the investigational treatments) [6]. The placebo response was found to be increased in recent RCTs assessing the efficacy of antiepileptic drugs [7], probably on account of misdiagnosis by less experienced investigators. This bias may be even greater in multicenter studies where the poor validity of the diagnosis is associated with a poor reliability due to suboptimal agreement among investigators. In order to maximize the validity and reliability of the diagnostic process, educational approaches and testing interrater reliability are recommended.

Problems may also arise when dealing with clinical conditions characterized by episodic occurrence. In the field of epilepsy, until recently the diagnosis had been made on the basis of two or more unprovoked seizures. In 2005, however, the International League against Epilepsy (ILAE) issued a new definition according to which the diagnosis of epilepsy could be made even at the presence of a single unprovoked seizure provided that a sustained tendency to relapse could be confirmed [8]. This tendency has been recently quantified as a 60% recurrence rate over 10 years [9]. A definition like this might have a strong influence on treatment effects, especially if patients with isolated seizures and patients with repeated seizures have an unbalanced distribution between treatment arms. This problem can only be solved by using strict inclusion and exclusion criteria. Similar detrimental effects may be present when diagnosing multiple sclerosis in patients with two or more relapses in different central nervous system areas and also in patients with a single episode and several demyelinating lesions on magnetic resonance imaging, in conformance with the most recent definitions of the disease [10].

Randomization Process

Randomization of patients in two or more treatment arms is the principal method to minimize selection bias. The random allocation fulfils the technical requirements: the reduction of selection bias, the production of balanced comparisons, and the quantification of errors attributable to chance. Randomization is effective because it guarantees that both known and unknown baseline differences across treatment groups are attributable to chance. While in large RCTs selection bias can be minimized, the same is not true for studies dealing with small samples. Randomization in blocks is a simple constraint improving balance among treatment groups. A block comprises a prespecified number of treatment assignments and must be a multiple of the number of treatment groups. Within each block, the order of treatment is randomly permuted but exactly balanced. In addition, as indicated above, stratification can be added to blocking to balance clinically important prognostic factors. In multicenter studies, blocking and stratification may be affected by the number of patients to be recruited by each individual center. For this reason, the size of each block should be defined based on the sustainability of recruitment by each center and a predefined number of patients should be enrolled by each center to account for a balanced distribution of patients with similar characteristics and outcome in experimental and control arms. Adaptive randomization procedures, like minimization, could be used in the event of inconstant treatment assignment. As RCTs for rare diseases are more likely to opt for the involvement of several centers, plans for randomization should consider these possible sources of bias before defining the extent of the stratification and blocking procedures.

Blinding

A blinding procedure helps to control assessment bias. Blinding may overcome positive and negative expectations of patients and investigators about treatment effects. Blinding may be single (the patient or, less frequently, the investigator), double (both the patient and the investigator), or triple (the patient, the investigator in charge of the treatment, and the person assigned to assess the response to treatment). Although, to preserve blinding, the investigational treatment and the comparator are shaped as to look, feel, and taste the same, the adverse effects of a treatment may not be entirely masked. This is the case, for example, with interferons for the treatment of multiple sclerosis. Flu-like symptoms are common in patients receiving interferons [11] and, despite the concurrent use of nonsteroidal anti-inflammatory agents, they may lead to unmasking experimental treatment. The gastrointestinal symptoms following the administration of cholinesterase inhibitors are another example [12].

The Choice of the End Points

The end points of an RCT represent the measures of treatment efficacy. Ideally, each end point should be objective, measurable, and clinically relevant. The efficacy of a treatment is better estimated by a quantitative assessment to be translated into a measurable difference. Unfortunately, this is not the case for several end points used in neurological disorders. Outcome measures may be represented by scales with variables represented by counts, categories, and event times. All these measures may or may not have a clinical significance to be transferred to the physician's desk. For example, the efficacy of drugs given for the prophylaxis of migraine is measured by the number of headache-free days, and comparisons between experimental treatment and a comparator are made counting the mean number of event-free days in the different treatment groups. This end point prevents the caring physician from making his/her personal judgment on the effects of treatment in each individual patient. Group means may be driven by outliers and find significant differences in spite of a lack of efficacy of the investigational treatment in the majority of patients. Even the use of categorical variables, like attaining a 50% or higher reduction in the baseline frequency of headache in each patient, may be biased by the number of headache attacks at study entry. More robust variables, like hospitalizations (epilepsy), admissions in nursery homes (Alzheimer's disease), or deaths (ALS) may be difficult to use because they may occur rarely in the course of the trial. Combinations of these end points can be used in the context of composite scores (as in patients with risk factors of stroke) but, again, the clinical significance of these variables is difficult to assess.

In several cases, surrogate end points are used. For example, the efficacy of a disease-modifying agent in multiple sclerosis can be assessed more easily when tested on the number of central nervous system lesions. Although surrogate end points increase the efficiency of RCTs, they cannot replace clinically relevant end points when assessing the efficacy of a treatment.

Clinical versus Statistical Significance

The measure of the effects of an investigational treatment is represented by the significance of the difference in the impact on prespecified end points between the experimental and the control arm. This difference must be statistically significant in order to overcome the play of chance. In this regard, the larger the sample size, the higher the chance for a difference to become statistically significant. This finding explains why in RCTs involving large numbers of patients the detection of statistically significant differences is not infrequent even if these differences are modest, i.e. clinically nonsignificant. For example, the efficacy of riluzole for the treatment of ALS was confirmed in a trial enrolling about 1,000 patients [13], and in this sample a statistically significant difference in the number of deaths during follow-up was found, which translated into a 3-month greater survival of the affected individuals. The choice of a prespecified clinically significant difference is thus required at the planning stage to demonstrate that a statistically significant effect of an investigational treatment is also clinically relevant.

Duration of the Experiment

For practical and economic purposes, an RCT must have a limited duration. In order to preserve the compliance with the study treatment, reduce the dropout rate, contain the costs, and at the same time show some treatment effects, the patients should be followed for a minimum period of time during which the chosen end point has at a least moderate probability to occur in the experimental and control arms. In neurological

diseases characterized by the recurrence of key events (e.g. headache, epilepsy, multiple sclerosis), symptoms should recur at a frequency sufficient for the event to be captured during the course of the experiment. As all these clinical conditions are heterogeneous in terms of severity (generally marked by a differing frequency of event occurrence), it follows that only the more severe disease varieties are represented in RCTs. Along with the selection of the study population, the duration of a trial, in order to preserve the internal validity and confirm the effects of treatment while adjusting for confounding variables, may not extend the results to all the potential recipients of the experimental treatment. In patients with progressing clinical conditions, the rate of progression may not uncover changes in the disease course which could be captured in the time frame of the experiment. The investigator may thus be forced to use end points sensitive to change in a short time period and refer once again to more severe disease varieties which may not represent all the patients affected by the same disease.

Adverse Treatment Events

The impact of an investigational treatment on the course of a disease must be assessed not only in terms of efficacy, but also in terms of safety and tolerability. In other words, a drug with a poor tolerability profile may not be useful even if proven significantly efficacious. On the other side, well-tolerated drugs can be marketed only if they are found to have a positive impact on the course of a disease. The problem of tolerability (and ease of use) of a drug has become of paramount importance in the last decades as better designed molecules have been developed, which has had an impact on the tolerability profile and interaction with other drugs. This is the case with several clinical conditions (neurological and nonneurological). Epilepsy is a typical example. The development of second- and third-generation compounds did not bring more effective drugs to the market, but did increase the availability of products with less adverse effects and interactions. However, as the tolerability profile of a drug heavily depends on the daily dose, the use of a suboptimal daily dose of a comparator (in this case, a dose higher than that usually administered in clinical practice) may give rise to results favoring the experimental product.

Internal versus External Validity

The results of an RCT must be assessed in terms of internal and external validity. The internal validity is the likelihood that the results are true and, as such, are supported by a robust study design. The external validity is the extent to which the results are applicable to those affected by the disease object of the trial. These two characteristics are to some extent opposites. Thus, a good experiment should be designed in order to satisfy both requirements. Regulatory trials are designed to enforce internal validity to provide unequivocal evidence of treatment efficacy. This is usually done at the expense of external validity. In contrast, pragmatic trials (i.e. trials performed to complement the results of regulatory trials) tend to privilege external validity, but in doing so they are supported by designs open to bias and, in this regard, their results are open to differing explanations. Both regulatory and pragmatic trials are thus needed to complete the efficacy, tolerability, and safety profile of a given treatment.

Alternative Design Models

A classical clinical trial cannot: (1) assess combined therapies, (2) take historical data into account, (3) safeguard ethics and efficacy during the course of long-term trials, (4) study drugs before well-established toxicity information is available, (5) account for the possibility of therapeutic equivalence between test and reference treatment, (6) study multiple treatments in one trial, and (7) adjust change scores for baseline levels [14]. Alternative designs helpful for such purposes are, respectively: (1) factorial designs, (2) historical controls designs, (3) group-sequential interim analysis designs, (4) sequential designs for continuous monitoring, (5) therapeutic equivalence designs, (6) multiple crossover-periods/multiple parallel-groups design, and (7) increased precision designs through multivariate adjustment. The main problems include the increased risks of type I and type II errors and the loss of validity criteria.

In conclusion, the clinical trial is still the ideal study design to confirm the efficacy of an experimental treatment in improving patient outcomes and provide decision-makers, such as patients, providers, policy-makers, and payers, with information as to which interventions are most effective for specific types of patients. Since the number of treatment options for many conditions has increased, comparative information is needed to support informed treatment choices. Efficacy measures how well interventions, including drugs, work under ideal circumstances, while effectiveness examines how well interventions work in real-world settings, where patients may have more complex conditions. This practical focus of the clinical trial introduces unique requirements for the design and implementation of studies. Tradeoffs of validity, relevance, feasibility, and timeliness must be considered. These unique considerations lead to questions concerning the appropriateness of study designs and methods. Understanding which approach is best to use under which circumstances is a question of significant debate. In practice, each research approach has advantages and disadvantages, and the research approach should be selected based upon the specific features or characteristics of the study question.

References

1 Pupillo E, Messina P, Logroscino G, Beghi E; SLALOM Group: Long-term survival in amyotrophic lateral sclerosis: a population-based study. Ann Neurol 2014;75:287–297.
2 Lublin FD, Reingold SC, Cohen JA, et al: Defining the clinical course of multiple sclerosis: the 2013 revisions. Neurology 2014;83:278–286.
3 Shorvon SD, Goodridge DM: Longitudinal cohort studies of the prognosis of epilepsy: contribution of the National General Practice Study of Epilepsy and other studies. Brain 2013;136:3497–3510.
4 Miller D, Barkhof F, Montalban X, Thompson A, Filippi M: Clinically isolated syndromes suggestive of multiple sclerosis, part I: natural history, pathogenesis, diagnosis, and prognosis. Lancet Neurol 2005;4:281–288.
5 Gilhus NE, Verschuuren JJ: Myasthenia gravis: subgroup classification and therapeutic strategies. Lancet Neurol 2015; 14:1023–1036.
6 Marson AG, Williamson PR, Clough H, Hutton JL, Chadwick DW; Epilepsy Monotherapy Trial Group: Carbamazepine versus valproate monotherapy for epilepsy: a meta-analysis. Epilepsia 2002;43:505–513.
7 Zaccara G, Giovannelli F, Schmidt D: Placebo and nocebo responses in drug trials of epilepsy. Epilepsy Behav 2015; 43:128–134.
8 Fisher RS, van Emde Boas W, Blume W, Elger C, Genton P, Lee P, Engel J Jr: Epileptic seizures and epilepsy: definitions proposed by the International League Against Epilepsy (ILAE) and the International Bureau for Epilepsy (IBE). Epilepsia 2005;46:470–472.
9 Fisher RS, Acevedo C, Arzimanoglou A, et al: ILAE official report: a practical clinical definition of epilepsy. Epilepsia 2014;55:475–482.
10 Polman CH, Reingold SC, Banwell B, et al: Diagnostic criteria for multiple sclerosis: 2010 revisions to the McDonald criteria. Ann Neurol 2011;69:292–302.
11 Galetta SL, Markowitz C: US FDA-approved disease-modifying treatments for multiple sclerosis: review of adverse effect profiles. CNS Drugs 2005;19:239–252.
12 Buckley JS, Salpeter SR: A risk-benefit assessment of dementia medications: systematic review of the evidence. Drug Aging 2015;32:453–467.
13 Lacomblez L, Bensimon G, Leigh PN, Guillet P, Meininger V: Dose-ranging study of riluzole in amyotrophic lateral sclerosis. Amyotrophic Lateral Sclerosis/Riluzole Study Group II. Lancet 1996; 347:1425–1431.
14 Cleophas TJ, Zwinderman AH: Limitations of randomized clinical trials. Proposed alternative designs. Clin Chem Lab Med 2000;38:1217–1223.

Ettore Beghi, MD
Laboratory of Neurological Disorders, IRCCS-Mario Negri
Institute for Pharmacological Research, Via Giuseppe La Masa 19
IT–20156 Milan (Italy)
E-Mail ettore.beghi@marionegri.it

Beghi E, Logroscino G (eds): The Right Therapy for Neurological Disorders. From Randomized Trials to Clinical Practice.
Front Neurol Neurosci. Basel, Karger, 2016, vol 39, pp 8–23 (DOI: 10.1159/000445409)

Peculiarities of Neurological Disorders and Study Designs

Ettore Beghi · Elisabetta Pupillo · Giorgia Giussani

Laboratory of Neurological Disorders, IRCCS-Mario Negri Institute for Pharmacological Research, Milan, Italy

Abstract

Background: Neurological disorders are heterogeneous clinical conditions with variable course and outcome. ***Summary:*** The basic aspects of the commonest neurological disorders are addressed along with the proposed structure of randomized clinical trials (RCTs). Dementing disorders, including Alzheimer's disease (AD), are clinical conditions in which altered cognitive functions are associated with behavioral and personality changes. Parkinson's disease (PD) is a multisystem disorder characterized by motor dysfunction associated with dysautonomia, sleep and olfactory disturbances, cognitive changes, and depression. Amyotrophic lateral sclerosis (ALS) is an invariably fatal clinical condition involving motor neurons. The available treatments are purely symptomatic for PD but virtually ineffective for AD and ALS. Headache disorders, multiple sclerosis, and epilepsy, three diseases characterized by recurrent symptoms and chronic or episodic course, can be fairly easily controlled by current treatments, but cannot be prevented nor cured. The objectives of treatments of neurodegenerative disorders include primary prevention, slowing or arrest of disease progression, and control of symptoms. Stroke is an acute clinical condition causing frequent disability and death, with only one approved treatment. There are many challenges to acute stroke clinical trials; among them, the very short therapeutic window and the issue of stroke heterogeneity. In this chapter, only the core elements of the study designs are outlined. ***Key Messages:*** The design of an RCT must be adapted to the basic characteristics of each clinical condition. © 2016 S. Karger AG, Basel

Neurological disorders are heterogeneous clinical conditions with variable course and outcome. Some of them are represented by acute monophasic entities with complete, partial, or no regression to baseline. Others are characterized by repeated episodes with return to the baseline conditions or, less frequently, with superimposed progression and accumulating disability. Others again have a relentless course with progressive worsening, albeit at differing speeds. All these peculiarities have a strong influence on the effects of treatments. For these reasons, the design of a randomized clinical trial (RCT) must be adapted to the basic characteristics of each clinical condition. In this chapter, the basic aspects of the commonest neurological disorders are addressed along with the proposed structure of RCTs. Only the core elements of the study designs will be outlined. A more comprehensive discussion of the characteristics of each disease can be found in the subsequent chapters. Those who are interested in having more information on the aims and structure of RCTs for selected neurological conditions are encouraged to read the guidelines on medicinal products issued by the European Medicines Agency (EMA) (http://emea.europa.eu) and the Iuphar Compendium of Basic Principles for Pharmacological Research in Humans (www.iuphar.org) that inspired the contents of this chapter.

Alzheimer's Disease and Other Dementias

Dementing disorders are a variety of clinical conditions characterized by progressive loss of cognitive functions, including memory, orientation, and language, and changes in personality and behavior. The commonest cause of dementia in the elderly is Alzheimer's disease (AD), followed by vascular dementia [1]. These two disorders partly overlap and can be considered the two extremes of a spectrum [2]. Other distinct forms of dementia include frontotemporal dementia, Parkinson's disease (PD) with dementia, dementia with Lewy bodies, and dementia associated with Huntington's disease. Each of them requires distinct diagnostic criteria [3]. Dementia may rarely occur in other clinical conditions including traumatic brain injury, schizophrenia, multiple sclerosis (MS), Creutzfeldt-Jakob disease, toxic and metabolic encephalopathies, and central nervous system (CNS) infections [3]. The diagnosis of dementia remains primarily clinical. Dementia must be distinguished from mild cognitive impairment (MCI), a memory complaint, preferably corroborated by an informant, with selective impairment of short-term memory but no substantial interference with daily living activities [4]. MCI lies between normal cognition and dementia, and is a risk factor for dementia. Dementing disorders are characterized by an increasing disability resulting in social and occupational decline.

The objectives of the treatment of dementia are manifold and include the primary prevention of the disease, slowing or arrest of cognitive decline, and improvement or abatement of behavioral symptoms. Data on the prevention of dementia are very limited because prevention studies must be necessarily large and prolonged, with expected high dropout rates. At present there is no treatment that modifies the natural history of the disease or changes its outcome. Potential treatments include drugs that increase the levels of neurotransmitters involved in cognitive functions, protect structurally or functionally damaged neurons, and replace neurons (neuronal regeneration).

Cholinesterase inhibitors (donepezil, rivastigmine, and galantamine) are the only drugs with some efficacy and a fairly acceptable tolerability profile [5]. However, these drugs tend to improve cognitive functions, activities of daily living, and behavior to a very limited extent and for a limited period of time. Memantine, an NMDA-receptor antagonist, in combination with cholinesterase inhibitors, is thought to have beneficial effects [6]. *Ginkgo biloba* has also been reported to be effective [7]. In contrast, progress in basic science and molecular biology has fostered new interest in symptomatic treatments and disease-modifying approaches.

The results of RCTs in dementing disorders must be interpreted in the light of methodological limitations, especially concerning the diagnostic criteria, disease stages, and definition and choice of the appropriate outcome. The typical design is a randomized, double-blind, placebo-controlled, parallel-group study comparing change at two primary end points, one of them reflecting the cognitive domain and the other reflecting the functional domain of impairment [8]. The ideal outcome should be easy to measure, and easily collectable at each follow-up over a significant period of time (ideally for several years). These measures should have good reliability, especially considering that many trials are multi-institutional.

Cognitive decline is difficult to quantify with the available instruments. Typical problems are floor and ceiling effects, regression to the mean, learning, and placebo effects. Moreover, the expected changes over a short period are small compared to the possible cognitive range of each scale. More suitable and robust end points include loss of independence, loss of specific daily living functions, and placement in a nursing home. However, these end points require prolonged follow-up and may be influenced by other environmental factors like the presence of an active caregiver, and the economic and social environment. In addition, several prognostic variables must be taken into account. These include, among others, the severity of dementia at admission, the apolipoprotein E genotype, the profile of β-amyloid and tau in the cerebrospinal fluid, and vascular risk factors.

Cognitive functions can be assessed with a battery of tests covering memory, language, constructional abilities, attention/concentration, and psychomotor speed. Remote and recent memory are explored along with recall and recognition for various modalities. Verbal and visuospatial memory are also investigated. The Mini-Mental State Examination (MMSE) [9] is generally used as a screening test for cognitive impairment while the Clinical Dementia Rating (CDR) [10] is used for grading disease severity. The Alzheimer's Disease Assessment Scale cognitive subscale (ADAS-cog) [11] is a comprehensive cognitive scale. However, none of the available instruments can be preferred as being more valid and reliable. Several scales have been proposed to measure the activities of daily living and to assess an overall clinical improvement, but none is preferably used in RCTs. Moreover, these tests have acceptable validity and reliability only in AD.

Depending on the type and course of each dementing disorder and the type of treatment, the duration of an RCT may vary from 6 months to several years. As there are no ideal study designs showing unambiguously a disease-modifying effect of a drug, long-term placebo-controlled studies are needed with periodic measurements of clinical outcomes to establish clinically relevant effects. This procedure, however, is not without problems. An RCT in patients with MCI should be of sufficient length for the primary end point (time to the conversion to dementia) to occur. As patients with MCI are expected to convert to dementia at a 10–15% rate per year [12], a statistically significant, clinically relevant, and sustained treatment effect can be documented only in a 3-year trial. Placebo must be used to detect the effects of treatment on disease progression. However, the study population enrolled in such a trial may have a high dropout rate for lack of compliance or premature mortality. In addition, patients with MCI may have the disease already at baseline, and thus the study is not really designed for prevention of dementia.

One critical issue is the incorporation of biomarkers (e.g. magnetic resonance imaging (MRI), positron emission tomography, cerebrospinal fluid markers) as surrogate end points. Biomarkers could signal the pathophysiology of the dementing condition, thus helping to differentiate disease-modifying from symptomatic effects. However, to be accepted, a biomarker should ideally respond to treatment, predict clinical response, and be correlated to the underlying pathophysiological processes. In this regard, each biomarker should be validated prior to being included in an RCT.

Parkinson's Disease

Parkinson's disease (PD) is the second most common neurodegenerative disorder in the elderly. The primary areas of CNS injury are typically the substantia nigra and the locus coeruleus. The disease is characterized by degeneration selective loss of dopaminergic neurons and, to a lesser extent, of other neural cells involving different neurotransmitter systems in different areas of the nervous system [13]. PD causes progressive disability, mostly characterized by motor dysfunction and including dysautonomia (sialorrhea, seborrhea, constipation, micturition disturbances, sexual dysfunction, orthostatic hypotension, hyperhidrosis), sleep and olfactory disturbances, cognitive changes (ranging from loss of executive function, or Lewy-body dementia, to a dementia indistinguishable from AD), and depression. The diagnosis of PD is clinical and requires bradykinesia and tremor, rigidity, and/or postural instability (at least 1 of these) [14]. PD must be differentiated from parkinsonian syndromes ('atypical' parkinsonisms) that include progressive supranuclear palsy, multiple system atrophy, and toxic, drug-induced and post-encephalitic parkinsonism [13]. There is neither a known cure nor any recognized method for slowing the ongoing degenerative process.

Currently available therapies include L-DOPA (combined with a peripheral DOPA-decarboxylase inhibitor), dopamine agonists, monoamine oxidase inhibitors, catecholamine-O-methyl transferase inhibitors, and anticholinergics [15]. These treatments are symptomatic and tend to minimize the motor dysfunction of PD through increase of the activity of the nigrostriatal dopamine system, although the overall benefit is partial, and not sustained over the years. In addition, these therapies have disabling and/or dose-limiting adverse effects. Acute adverse effects include nausea and hypotension. Chronic adverse effects include involuntary movements (dyskinesia, dystonia, choreoathetosis), somnolence, psychiatric symptoms (hallucinations, delusions, psychosis), and autonomic side effects. Treatments for the nonmotor disabilities of PD are few, and none are universally effective. In contrast to PD, there are no effective therapies for 'atypical' parkinsonisms, although existing antiparkinsonian therapies may provide short-lived partial benefit for a minority of patients. The response to some antiparkinsonian agents, notably those including L-DOPA, can vary dramatically over time. Variation can occur over hours or even minutes during the course of a single dose, and can be further modified by the time of day, number of prior doses, type of concurrent therapies, and timing and protein content of meals. Similarly, the adverse effects of antiparkinsonian therapies, such as dyskinesias, typically wax and wane during the course of a day.

The majority of antiparkinsonian agents have been tested comparing active treatment to placebo. Experimental drugs have rarely been compared to existing therapies. In addition, the effects of existing therapies within clinical subgroups, defined by age, gender, or race/ethnicity, or by clinical phenotype, are virtually unknown. Little is known regarding the benefit of any therapeutic agent for prolonged periods of time. Two trials (DATATOP and UKPDRG) followed patients for up to 10 years with only the latter being designed to test differences in mortality [16, 17].

The therapeutic regimen preventing the development of adverse effects or altering the course of disease remains unknown. Almost nothing is known regarding the effects of antiparkinsonian drugs on survival in PD.

As there is no diagnostic test for PD, there is a potential for diagnostic error especially during the first years of disease. In addition, most patients can function without therapy during the early course of the disease. Another obstacle is represented by the requirement for symptomatic therapy at the onset of disabling symptoms, which implies the need to test any experimental drug as an adjunct to an established therapy because comparison to placebo alone would not be ethical. However, comparison of a new drug to placebo is appropriate for patients treated for the first time (sometimes called de novo patients), and this design is preferred by both the Food and

Drug Administration (FDA) and the EMA for new drugs intended for registration as monotherapy. In this special setting, provision for 'rescue' with a symptomatic agent may be advisable.

European regulatory authorities recommend using different designs depending on the objectives of the study [18]. These include symptomatic treatments, therapies aimed to modify disease progression and/or late motor complications, therapies aimed to delay disease progression and/or late motor fluctuations, and therapies aimed to replace neural loss.

RCTs testing symptomatic drugs in early PD before L-DOPA (de novo patients) should be randomized double-blind placebo-controlled, and of at least 6-month duration. In addition to the placebo arm, an active control arm should be included in the design to show a favorable benefit/risk ratio of the experimental drug as compared to a gold standard. The choice of the comparator and the dose should be justified. RCTs in patients with motor symptoms and/or motor fluctuations while receiving L-DOPA should be double-blind, placebo-controlled, add-on trials of at least 3-month duration, in which L-DOPA and any other relevant treatments should be kept constant at the best tolerable dose. Superiority should be demonstrated against placebo and eventually also against the active comparator. In these studies, end points should be the improvement of motor symptoms (including motor complications) and activities of daily living. The UPDRS II (activities of daily living) and the UPDRS III (motor examination) are acceptable scales to assess motor function in PD as having satisfactory validity and reliability [19].

RCTs of drugs aimed to modify disease progression should also be add-on, double-blind, and placebo-controlled; however, in order to detect disease-modifying effects, the studies should be long term and with different end points according to the objectives. In studies on drugs aimed at postponing late motor complications, efficacy should be measured with actuarial methods (e.g. time to late motor complications). In RCTs on treatments aimed to delay disease progression, a definite milestone should be chosen as the primary end point. Milestones should vary depending on the severity and duration of the disease to reflect a substantial benefit in terms of improvement of motor impairment and functional disability. Relevant clinical end points include falls, cognitive impairment, loss of self-sufficiency, and nursing home placement. RCTs on the effects of treatments replacing neuronal loss are still in their infancy because cell therapy in PD is confined to the experimental stage. Robust safety studies and trials demonstrating that a critical mass of grafted neurons are alive and functional when correctly placed are awaited.

Biomarkers measuring cerebral dopamine uptake, single-photon emission computed tomography-β-CIT, or dopamine receptor density (positron emission tomography-F-DOPA) cannot be used as surrogate biomarkers since a correlation with the clinical function is as yet unproven [20, 21]. The lack of correlation between the effects of a drug on the worsening of symptoms and on other measures of disease progression prevents any contention that the drug is a disease modifier.

Headache

Headache disorders are a relevant source of disability and costs for the individual and at a population level [22–24]. The two commonest headache varieties include migraine and tension-type headache. Migraine manifests in attacks ranging from a few hours to 3 days [22]. Two main types of migraine are distinguished, migraine with aura and without aura. In migraine with aura the headache is preceded by reversible neurological symptoms. Because migraine affects people particularly during their productive years, its economic impact is high. Tension-type headache is the most common headache disorder. Most tension-type headaches are episodic, with occasional attacks lasting hours. In its chronic and much more disabling subtype, a tension-type headache may occur several days a week and overlaps with other headache forms. Cluster headache is less common and, contrary to migraine and tension-type headache, affects men more than women. Typically occurring in bouts, cluster headache is characterized by frequent short-lasting but excruciating unilateral localized frontal or periorbital pain, accompanied by similarly localized autonomic symptoms. In the rarer chronic subtype, there are no periods of remission.

Symptomatic treatments (analgesics and antiemetics) are still the mainstay for acute migraine therapy [25]. They are also the first-line treatments for tension-type headache [26]. Triptans, a separate category of drugs made available in the last decades for the acute treatment of migraine, are efficacious in several patients not responding to other analgesics and are of limited value for cluster headache [25, 27]. Triptans are not always efficacious and not universally tolerated. Current research is mostly focused on head-to-head comparisons between triptans, invariably showing minor differences, and prevents development of new drugs with different mechanisms of action. For all primary headache disorders, the currently available prophylactic drugs are, at best, of limited value. The agents used for migraine prophylaxis include β-blockers, calcium blockers, antiepileptic drugs (AEDs), methysergide and other antiserotonin agents, and tricyclic antidepressants.

The experimental plan for the assessment of an investigational drug for the treatment of headache includes separate designs for drugs used for the treatment of the headache attack and for prophylactic compounds. The diagnostic criteria are those of the International Headache Society (IHS) [28]. Patients to be included should have had migraine for at least 1 year with a 3-month retrospective history. A prophylactic treatment, where present, should have remained unchanged for 3 months prior to inclusion. Prophylaxis is justified when attacks occur at least 2 times per month.

If prophylaxis is withdrawn, 1 month or longer should elapse prior to inclusion. There should be at least 48 h of freedom from pain between attacks. The measurement scales used should be justified and validated for migraine. The primary end point for a drug given to abort an attack should be the percent of patients free of pain at 2 h. The primary end point for headache prophylaxis should be the frequency of attacks within a prespecified period.

Candidate drugs must be firstly assessed for efficacy against placebo. For drugs for the acute treatment of migraine, pharmacokinetic studies should be conducted during the attack because absorption may be delayed by gastric stasis. For this reason, oral administration may not be ideal and alternative routes may be required in patients complaining of nausea and vomiting. In addition, rapid bioavailability is needed for treatment to be effective, and this is unlikely to be achieved by the oral route. Typical studies should be double-blind, with parallel groups comparing one or more doses. Three-arm trials are required for internal validation in active comparator studies because of a large and highly variable placebo effect. Alternatively, therapeutic efficacy may be tested in superiority trials against a well-established comparator.

The superiority of the test agent in comparison with placebo should be convincingly demonstrated in randomized, two-armed double-blind controlled parallel group prophylactic trials. Prophylactic trials should allow time for dose titration and time for efficacy to develop and be measurable. This may require 3–6 months of follow-up depending on the severity and frequency of attacks. The objectives of treatment vary in migraine and tension-type headache. Migraine prophylaxis is intended to reduce the frequency of attacks while in chronic tension-type headache the intent is to induce reversion to the episodic subtype. In patients with cluster headache, prophylaxis should ideally prevent the occurrence of a cluster period. However, in episodic cluster headache, spontaneous remission of the cluster period may attenuate a trial's ability to detect true treatment benefits. Appropriate acute therapy must be allowed for individual attacks.

Phase III pivotal RCTs are randomized double-blind trials incorporating one or more doses of a study drug according to the findings of phase II trials. They must preferably use parallel groups. For acute and prophylactic therapy, phase III trials should include active comparators. Pivotal acute-treatment trials should also address the consistency of the therapeutic response across multiple attacks. In this regard, in migraine and episodic tension-type headache, long-term follow-up studies are advisable. These trials also contribute to safety evaluation.

As the headache may reach the peak at differing times, with subsequent spontaneous resolution, phase III trials should also explore the relationship between timing of acute treatment and effect. Such studies in migraine with aura should include treatment during the aura phase.

RCTs in migraine and episodic tension-type headache should consider the use of rescue medications as indirect measures of treatment efficacy. Prophylactic trials require a minimum of 3 months of treatment for migraine or chronic tension-type headache, but longer periods (4–6 months or more) would be desirable.

In all primary headache disorders, treatment safety is a major concern since the disorders themselves are frequently mild and/or self-limiting. This is particularly true when using drugs with teratogenic potential in women of childbearing age [29]. On the other hand, given the high prevalence of these diseases, a wide population (not always represented by the patients included in RCTs) will be exposed to drugs marketed for headache. Postmarketing studies are awaited and special studies are required in selected diseased populations. In this regard, special protocols are needed for children, whose needs may be different, and for the elderly, who are more at risk of symptomatic headache as well as comorbidities.

Epilepsy

Epilepsy is a fairly common chronic neurological disease affecting both sexes and all ages, with peaks in the two extremes and a slight predominance in males [30, 31]. The disease, defined by the occurrence of two unprovoked seizures, one unprovoked seizure at high risk of recurrence, or an epilepsy syndrome [32], is the complication of a spectrum of disorders and injuries to the CNS, documented in about one half of cases and mostly represented by cerebrovascular disorders, traumatic brain injuries, tumors, developmental or degenerative disorders, infections, and genetic defects [33]. Up to 85% of patients achieve seizure remission immediately after treatment start or at different times during the course of the disease, with the remaining 15% being truly drug-resistant cases [34, 35]. Despite its favorable outcome with the available treatments, epilepsy represents a relevant socioeconomic burden. In newly diagnosed patients, a satisfactory response to the initial treatment can positively affect the early prognosis of the disease [34]. However, the long-term outcome of epilepsy is apparently unaffected by early treatment. Early remission only indicates that the disease runs a mild course, which is predicted by seizure control after treatment start. However, more recent studies done on the long-term prognosis of epilepsy found that seizure outcome is more complex and follows differing patterns [35]. The course of the disease can be predicted by the response to early treatment only in some cases, and five main patterns can be recognized. These include early remission within the first year of treatment continuing to terminal remission, late remission after the first year of treatment continuing to terminal remission, a relapsing-remitting course which reenters remission following a relapse after an early or late remission, a worsening course that does not reenter remission following a relapse after an early or late remission, and no remission at any time. Thus, drug-resistant epilepsy can be better interpreted as a dynamic process, predicted by patient and disease characteristics, timing, and type of drug.

Epilepsy in childhood differs in part from epilepsy in adults because different seizure types may occur depending on the level of maturity of the brain and due to the occurrence of seizures as part of age-dependent epilepsy syndromes [36]. An epilepsy syndrome may persist or change in characteristics over time. Moreover, epilepsy may affect the normal development of children in the broadest sense. In the elderly, RCTs should consider the increased susceptibility to adverse effects, with special reference to cognitive functions, vigilance, and cardiovascular system, and pharmacokinetic and/or pharmacodynamic interactions with other drugs used to treat comorbidities.

Most AEDs have been tested and found to be effective against focal seizures with or without secondary generalization. Some AEDs show a broader spectrum of efficacy, while for others efficacy is limited to selected seizure types (e.g. absence seizures). In terms of epilepsy syndromes, it is important to know which (and how) seizure types associated with a given syndrome are affected by a specific medication. In addition, some AEDs are contraindicated because they may exacerbate some seizure types.

For most AEDs the knowledge of their spectrum of effectiveness is limited as most clinical trials have been performed in patients with focal seizures with or without secondary generalization. In addition, inclusion of patients in trials has usually been based on seizure type and not on epilepsy syndrome.

In this complex scenario, any investigational treatment must be assessed for efficacy using a two-step process and two different study designs. The first step is represented by add-on parallel-group placebo-controlled trials in which the drug is tested in patients receiving the best available drugs (no more than two or three compounds) and drug schedules. Patients with drug-resistant epilepsy are enrolled and followed for 6 months on average. Depending on the FDA and the EMA requirements, the primary end points include the percent change in seizure frequency during the treatment phase compared to baseline and, respectively, the responder rate, i.e. the percentage of patients with a greater than 50% reduction in seizure frequency compared to baseline. Unfortunately, the antiepileptic action of a new drug cannot be fully assessed in an add-on trial because concomitant drugs may interfere for a number of reasons (e.g. pharmacokinetic and/or pharmacodynamic interactions, additive toxic effects). These changes cannot be disentangled from the true effects of the investigational treatment. The interaction potential may affect both the experimental drug and the concomitant treatments, resulting in increased or decreased effects and, at the same time, increased or decreased adverse effects.

The second step refers to the assessment of the investigational drug as monotherapy. For ethical reasons, in these studies the investigational drug must be compared to an active compound, which in theory should be the best available treatment. The only possibility to use placebo in a monotherapy trial refers to short-term RCTs in which conversion to monotherapy is tried. Although escape criteria are used to minimize the risks (e.g. the patient is withdrawn after a certain number of seizures), these trials should not be performed. Thus, in these studies, patients with newly diagnosed epilepsy are the main target. The preferred design is the superiority trial, in which the research hypothesis is that the investigational compound is better than the comparator. Noninferiority monotherapy trials have also been considered to investigate products which, in spite of a noninferior efficacy profile, are better tolerated and easier to use in terms of pharmacokinetic characteristics and lack of drug-drug interactions. However, this design should be not encouraged to prevent the development of 'me-too' drugs. The minimum duration of the study is 12 months. The primary end point is the achievement of seizure freedom, measured as the time to the first (or second) seizure.

The design of RCTs in epilepsy must be in line with the peculiarities of the disease. As epilepsy is characterized by repeated unpredictable events, the epileptic seizures, eligible patients for add-on placebo-controlled trials must be represented by individuals with seizures possibly occurring in a limited time period. Patients with drug-resistant epilepsy and, among them, individuals with frequent seizures, are thus preferred. In addition, experimental drugs are tested preferably in patients with the commonest epilepsy varieties. Except for studies done in children with focal epilepsy, with absence of seizures, or with selected epilepsy syndromes (e.g. Lennox-Gastaut syndrome), RCTs are rarely performed in pediatric populations. There are also few studies done in the elderly and virtually no studies done in special diseased populations, such as patients with mental handicaps. In contrast, there are a number of pragmatic trials which have investigated selected therapeutic strategies, like treatment of the first seizure, discontinuation of treatment, or the comparative use of different AEDs in newly diagnosed patients or in patients in whom a first monotherapy failed. These trials are generally open-label and, when different drugs are compared, use retention time (i.e. time to drug withdrawal for lack of efficacy and/or adverse events) as a primary end point. Pragmatic trials are useful RCTs to complete the assessment of drug effectiveness in clinical practice. There are still several situations in the therapeutic process in epilepsy which require proper investigation with pragmatic trials. These include, among others, the comparative efficacy of some second- and third-generation compounds, the prevention of acute symptomatic seizures (i.e. seizures occurring in close temporal relation with acute structural, toxic, or metabolic CNS insults) [37] and unprovoked seizures, the minimum target dose in newly diagnosed epilepsy, and the downtitration of drugs in long-term seizure-free patients.

Multiple Sclerosis

MS is a chronic inflammatory and degenerative disease affecting predominantly the white matter of the CNS [38]. The etiology of MS is unknown. MS is thought to be mediated by an autoimmune process triggered by an infection which is superimposed on a genetic predisposition. The revised McDonald criteria [39] incorporating MRI criteria for dissemination in time and space are widely accepted for the diagnosis of MS. MS affects most commonly young adults and predominates in females [38]. Environmental factors are virtually unknown and genetic factors involved with the regulatory mechanisms of the immune system have been only partly documented [40]. The symptoms of the disease tend to occur almost everywhere in the CNS, but the commonest sites of onset are the optic nerve, spinal cord, brainstem, and cerebellum [38]. The course of MS is heterogeneous and three main patterns have been described, the commonest being relapsing remitting, followed by secondary progressive and primary progressive [41, 42]. Relapses present subacute onset and duration ranging from days to weeks, followed by full remission or, less frequently, residual disability. Depending on the site of onset, the disease may present a differing tendency to recur and to present with an accumulating disability. The term 'clinically isolated syndrome' refers to a first clinical episode attributable to a demyelinating event complying with the diagnostic criteria for definite MS, i.e. dissemination of demyelinating events in time and space either observed clinically or radiographically [43]. The presence and the number of asymptomatic lesions is considered a risk factor for future relapses and brought MS experts to anticipate the diagnosis, which in the past was confirmed only by the occurrence of at least two attacks in two different sites and in two separate time periods [39]. These clinical pictures and patterns of disease course are evidence that MS has a wide clinical spectrum, represented, at one extreme, by a single episode with full remission during the lifetime and, at the other extreme, a progressive and devastating course with increasing disability and eventually anticipated death.

The current therapeutic approach to MS involves symptomatic treatment, treatment of acute relapses, and disease-modifying therapies. Symptomatic treatment refers to all therapies aimed at improving disease symptoms and complications, such as fatigue, spasticity, ataxia, walking disability, weakness, bladder and bowel disturbances, and cognitive impairment. These treatments are nonspecific. In contrast, MS-specific treatments are those that intend to interfere with the pathophysiology of the disease, facilitating remyelination or axonal conductivity. Time-limited courses of steroids (predominantly methylprednisolone) are given at the time of a relapse [44]. However, methylprednisolone shortens the duration of a relapse, but has no influence on its sequelae. To date, treatments have aimed to modify the course of the disease by suppressing or modulating the immune responses involved in MS pathogenesis. Therapeutic proteins and monoclonal antibodies have been approved for use in this therapeutic context [45]. These drugs have a broad range of targets including, among others, T-cell receptors, costimulation molecules, and chemokines. β-Interferons and glatiramer acetate are the first products found to affect the disease course by preventing relapses [46]. However, the effects of these drugs on residual disability are unproven. Therefore, an effect on disability cannot be claimed solely based on relapse prevention. Other, more promising molecules for their apparent effects on the progression of the disease include natalizumab (a monoclonal antibody) and fingolimod (a drug sequestering lymphocytes in lymph nodes) [47, 48]. These therapies aim to prevent relapses and ultimately intend to decrease the rate of accumulation of disability. Due to the risks of opportunistic infections, malignancies, and other systemic adverse drug reactions, several of these treatment options are considered as second-line options and should be restricted to patients with rapidly evolving MS or those who had a suboptimal response to prior therapies.

The design of RCTs in MS varies according to the disease spectrum and to the presence of active treatments in clinical practice. With reference to the study population, the change of the diagnostic criteria for MS has led to inclusion in RCTs of patients diagnosed earlier in the course of the disease. These patients tend to have a lower number of relapses as compared to patients recruited in studies performed over the last decades. Efficacy of experimental drugs should be established by means of randomized double-blind parallel-group trials. The preferred approach would be an RCT showing superiority of the experimental drug versus an active comparator (a β-interferon or glatiramer acetate, or, for acute relapses, methylprednisolone). The anticipated benefit-risk profile of the new product needs to be taken into account. This means that the expected benefit of treatment in consideration of disease activity should be weighed against the anticipated risk of opportunistic infections, malignancies, and other potential serious safety issues. Add-on study designs may be considered as an alternative only if there are no synergistic drug effects leading to increased safety concerns, e.g. a synergistic immunosuppressive effect. A useful design is a three-arm trial looking at superiority of the combination versus both products used as monotherapy [49].

Given the long-term use of an established drug therapy in MS, data on large and representative groups of patients for a sufficient period of time should be provided. As a major category of products used or tested in MS are considered to act as immunomodulators, special attention should be paid to autoimmune disorders and the tumor-facilitating/-inducing potential of these products. It may be need to address the risk of opportunistic infections and malignancies in postmarketing studies. A pregnancy register should be also considered.

At present, MRI measurements are not a validated surrogate end point for the clinical outcome and should not be used as a primary end point in pivotal studies evaluating new agents [49]. MRI findings are useful to test a potentially effective drug in proof-of-concept and dose-finding studies. In pivotal studies MRI is useful to test the consistency of imaging findings with the clinical effect. The contribution of neuroimaging to the anticipation of the diagnosis of MS in clinically isolated syndromes at high risk of relapse led the investigators to undertake an increasing number of trials in these syndromes with the intent of reducing the number of cases with relapses, i.e. converting to MS. These studies raise ethical concerns because, in spite of a virtual lack of evidence of any effect on the progression of the disease, an increasing number of patients who may not experience a clinical relapse are exposed to treatments that are sometimes poorly tolerated, expensive, and likely to expose patients to serious adverse events.

The presence of surrogate end points (e.g. asymptomatic lesions on MRI) has been accepted by regulatory agencies as markers of treatment efficacy in phase II trials while pivotal (phase III) trials must still rely on clinical end points. The latter are represented by the occurrence of relapses and the clinical measurement of the progression of disability. The primary efficacy parameters based on relapses include the annualized relapse rate and the time to the next relapse. The primary efficacy parameter for the progression of the disease should be a clinically measured delay of the progression of disability. The effects of treatment on relapses and disease progression should be both tested as a primary and a secondary end point depending on the aims of the study. The commonest scale used to measure disease progression is the Kurtzke Expanded Disability Status Scale (EDSS) [50]. Progression is measured by an increase of at least one full step on EDSS. The scale is, however, insensitive to short-term changes, is heavily weighted toward ambulation, and is not linear. Within each clinical form of the disease, relapse activity and severity of disability (e.g. defined according to an EDSS score of <3.5, 4–6, and >6.5) are important characteristics to define a priori subgroups of patients. Stratification for milder and more severely affected patients is recommended.

Placebo-controlled studies are still required to demonstrate treatment efficacy. However, the use of placebo raises ethical concerns because active treatments are available. For this reason, add-on placebo-controlled trials must be undertaken on top of standard treatments given at optimal regimens. As with trials done in other neurological disorders, patients experiencing frequent relapses are enrolled, which limits the external validity of the study. Even with this limitation, RCTs in MS must have a minimum duration of 2 years.

To evaluate the efficacy of an experimental drug against disability progression, only patients without a recent relapse but with evidence of recent progression independently of relapses should be included. This is needed to exclude possible effects of relapse activity on disability. However, occurrence of relapse activity needs to be assessed during the study and taken into account when determining a confirmed progression of disability. The duration of a study intended to demonstrate a clinically meaningful effect on relapses will depend on the activity of the population studied and in cases of a prevalent population with a milder disease course may need to last at least 3 years.

RCTs in MS may also address the treatment of specific symptoms or disease complications (e.g. cognitive impairment, motion and mobility, fatigue, pain, autonomic dysfunction). End points in these trials should include validated scales measuring specific neurological symptoms, pain, cognitive functions, and other patient-reported outcomes.

Biomarkers other than neuroimaging are currently unavailable that may identify subgroups at risk for rapid disease progression and/or patients that benefit more from treatment than others.

The usefulness of developing products for patients with a clinically isolated syndrome not to be classified as MS or inclusion of radiological isolated syndrome is considered doubtful [49].

Amyotrophic Lateral Sclerosis

Amyotrophic lateral sclerosis (ALS) is a severe clinical condition involving motor neurons and invariably leading to death within approximately 3–5 years from the onset of symptoms [51]. Although motor neuron damage has been attributed, among others, to oxidative damage, changes in intracellular calcium levels, glutamate excitoxicity, and genetic factors, the pathophysiology of ALS is still largely unknown, with emerging evidence of a complex interaction between genetic and environmental factors [52, 53]. The main clinical presentations of the disease include upper and lower motor neuron signs in the limbs and bulbar signs, presenting with speech and swallowing difficulties. Other, less common presentations include thoracic-abdominal (axial) involvement and respiratory involvement at onset. Primary lateral sclerosis (pure upper motor neuron involvement) and progressive muscular atrophy (pure lower motor neuron involvement) have slower progression and better prognosis and are not considered typical ALS [54]. The clinical spectrum of the disease is heterogeneous and the duration of the disease can be significantly affected by several prognostic indicators, including age, symptom progression, opening symptoms (bulbar or spinal), and degree of respiratory insufficiency [55].

Effective treatments for ALS have remained elusive. Only riluzole, a drug thought to affect glutamate metabolism, improves survival (albeit to a modest extent) [56]. Explanations for the negative results include a likely heterogeneity in disease susceptibility and pathogenic mechanisms, and defective design of published clinical trials. Better knowledge of the representativeness of the study populations, identification of the main prognostic predictors, and a critical appraisal of the study design and methods provide the basis for the implementation of more successful clinical trials.

The unbalanced distribution of these variables may affect the interpretation of the results when the efficacy of treatment is assessed in an RCT. The use of different outcome measures is another source of variability in the assessment of treatment effects. Mortality is the most valuable end point because it is not affected by the patient's or investigator's subjective judgment. However, mortality may not present to a significant extent in a short-term RCT, especially when dealing with incident cases and patients with slow symptom progression. By contrast, the use of all available measures of disability is likely to be confounded by disagreement among investigators on the outcome measures and the interpretation of findings. Tracheostomy, percutaneous gastrostomy and mechanical ventilation may vary according to the patient's and physician's judgment. Even the commonest disability scales, like electrophysiological findings and measures of health-related quality of life, involve different interpretations, which may be confounding elements in multicenter RCTs. Safety and tolerability of treatment must also be considered. The severity of ALS may justify the use of compounds with less-than-optimal tolerability, but this may not be acceptable when lifetime treatments are required and/or the death risk may be increased.

The primary goal of ALS treatment is the prevention or delay of disease progression (increased survival and delay or stabilization of disease progression). Symptomatic treatment must be also considered. Due to the variability of clinical findings early in the course of the disease and the lack of established biomarkers, early diagnosis of ALS can be difficult. Symptoms are often not recognized until considerable motor function has been lost and the mean delay in time from presentation to diagnosis is still approximately 1 year [57]. For this reason, the selection of a homogeneous study population early in the course of the disease might be difficult. However, where possible, study participants should be stratified according to known prognostic factors and time from first symptom to diagnosis. Only patients with definite or probable ALS according to the modified El Escorial criteria should be included in RCTs.

Survival time should be a primary end point of ALS trials aiming at disease modification. The ALS Functional Rating Scale (ALSFRS-R) [58] is the most widely used instrument to measure function in ALS patients. The ALSFRS-R is a validated disease-specific scale. Functional decline in untreated patients is expected to average about 1 point per month [59]. Measurement of muscle strength [60] and forced vital capacity are the most accepted secondary end points. Decrease in weight is a potentially useful additional indicator of muscle loss and disease progression.

The conventional design of RCTs in ALS is the double-blind randomized placebo-controlled trial. As riluzole is approved for modifying disease progression in ALS and is currently prescribed to the majority of patients, there are ethical concerns on doing placebo-controlled studies. RCTs should thus include riluzole as a comparator or as the background treatment. For add-on trials, patients stabilized on riluzole should be randomized to receive either the new drug or placebo. For a monotherapy indication, a two-arm parallel-group placebo-controlled trial could be performed in patients not taking riluzole for reasons unrelated to the trial. Trial duration should be at least 12 months.

Drugs authorized for improvement of ALS symptoms are as yet unavailable. Therefore, two-arm parallel-group placebo-controlled trials are still currently recommended. The main aim of the trial would be to demonstrate superiority to placebo. Studies on symptomatic drugs may be of shorter duration than for drugs with disease-modifying effects. Depending of the mechanism of action, pivotal efficacy trials of 3–6 months

duration could be sufficient [61]. Safety data over 12 months may be also required to exclude a negative impact on disease-modifying outcomes. This follow-up also allows estimating the duration of the symptomatic effect.

Stroke

Stroke is one of the leading causes of disability and death in the elderly in Western countries [62, 63]. Ischemic stroke is the commonest cause followed by hemorrhagic stroke and subarachnoid hemorrhage. The distinct pathophysiology and the clinical characteristics of these three entities imply three distinct therapeutic approaches.

The only approved acute stroke therapy is IV t-plasminogen activator [64]. Although numerous compounds have shown benefit in animal models of brain infarction, RCTs on neuroprotectants in acute ischemic stroke have always failed. There are many challenges to acute stroke clinical trials, including the very short therapeutic window and the issue of stroke heterogeneity. Stroke is a syndrome and only a very small percentage of all stroke patients present to hospitals in time to consider reperfusion therapy [64]. Many drugs have been tested in humans prematurely based on inadequate preclinical testing. Many trials have been seriously underpowered due to overly optimistic expectations, and the risk of brain hemorrhage has precluded aggressive multimodal treatment strategies. The prediction of vascular event rates in trial control arms is critical in designing clinical trials. Diagnostic technologies have evolved dramatically over the last 50 years and have altered events. The development of computed tomography (CT) and MRI has increased the diagnosis of incident strokes. There have been great discrepancies between the actual sample sizes used in clinical trials and the sample sizes that would have been required for adequately powered trials, based on actual observed event rates. The ratios of adequately powered sample sizes to the actual median values of trials were 35.4 in the 1960s, 29.3 in the 1970s, 12.5 in the 1980s, 9.2 in the 1990s, and 4.4 in the 2000s [65]. This improving trend indicates clinical trialists' increasing awareness of, and attention to, the problem of underpowered trials. However, the problem of needing very large sample sizes to adequately power trials is greater than in the past. More accurate prediction of vascular event rates in control arms is accordingly urgently needed.

The therapeutic goals in acute stroke are expected to improve functional outcome (in terms of independence in the management of daily living activities), improve neurological deficit, and ultimately prevent death. Several options are available for primary efficacy end points. These include the proportion of patients who regain functional independence after stroke and the proportion of survivors. Mortality can be also used as a safety parameter, as any new drug should be accepted for approval only if detrimental effects on survival can be reasonably excluded. Several scales are available for the measurement of stroke-related impairment and functional disability. These include, among others, the National Institute of Health Stroke Scale [66], the Scandinavian Stroke Scale [67], the Canadian Stroke Scale [68], and the Unified Stroke Scale [69]. In addition, functional outcome scales can be used. The most widely used measure of functional disability in stroke studies is the Barthel Index [70]. The Modified Rankin Scale [71] and the Glasgow Outcome Scale [72] are also used as overall measures of disability and handicap. These scales can be used not only as outcome measures, but also to stratify the patients in different categories with reference to the severity of the disease. An appropriate stratification may also be necessary if patients with mild or severe stroke types are to be excluded.

Depending on the claimed indication, patients with ischemic stroke and patients with hemorrhagic stroke should be the object of different RCTs. Diagnostic tests (CT and cerebrospinal fluid in patients with suspected subarachnoid hemorrhage with negative CT findings) are thus necessary to complement the clinical diagnosis.

Study populations should also be characterized with respect to stroke risk factors and comorbidities (and related treatments) in order to exclude individuals with functional disability related to other clinical conditions and to disentangle the effects of the investigational treatment from the effects of other known confounders.

As thrombolytic drugs are now the gold standard for the treatment of ischemic stroke, placebo-controlled studies should be performed only in patients receiving thrombolytic drugs. Monotherapy trials should be only performed using a thrombolytic agent as the active comparator. Regardless of the study design, an intention-to-treat analysis should be the primary statistical analysis.

The minimum duration of an RCT in stroke patients is 3–6 months. During this period, except for rescue medications, other treatments with potential impact on therapeutic outcome should be excluded or, where necessary, standardized. Interaction studies with drugs commonly used in this target population should be performed.

References

1 Rizzi L, Rosset I, Roriz-Cruz M: Global epidemiology of dementia: Alzheimer's and vascular types. Biomed Res Int 2014;2014:908915.
2 Attems J, Jellinger KA: The overlap between vascular disease and Alzheimer's disease – lessons from pathology. BMC Med 2014;12:206.
3 Sachdev PS, Blacker D, Blazer DG, et al: Classifying neurocognitive disorders: the DSM-5 approach. Nat Rev Neurol 2014;10:634–642.
4 Langa KM, Levine DA: The diagnosis and management of mild cognitive impairment: a clinical review. JAMA 2014; 312:2551–2561.
5 O'Brien JT, Burns A; BAP Dementia Consensus Group: Clinical practice with anti-dementia drugs: a revised (second) consensus statement from the British Association for Psychopharmacology. J Psychopharmacol 2011;25:997–1019.

6 Schmidt R, Hofer E, Bouwman FH, et al: EFNS-ENS/EAN Guideline on concomitant use of cholinesterase inhibitors and memantine in moderate to severe Alzheimer's disease. Eur J Neurol 2015;22: 889–898.

7 von Gunten A, Schlaefke S, Überla K: Efficacy of *Ginkgo biloba* extract EGb 761® in dementia with behavioural and psychological symptoms: a systematic review. World J Biol Psychiatry 2015: 1–12.

8 CPMP/EWP/553/95 Rev 1 (2008). www. ema.europa.eu/.../WC500133438.pdf.

9 Folstein MF, Folstein SE, McHugh PR: 'Mini-mental state'. A practical method for grading the cognitive state of patients for the physician. J Psychiatr Res 1975;12:189–198.

10 Morris JC: The Clinical Dementia Rating (CDR) – current version and scoring rules. Neurology 1993;43:2412–2414.

11 Rosen WG, Mohs RC, Davis KL: A new rating scale for Alzheimer's disease. Am J Psychiatry 1984;141:1356–1364.

12 Vega JN, Newhouse PA: Mild cognitive impairment: diagnosis, longitudinal course, and emerging treatments. Curr Psychiatry Rep 2014;16:490.

13 Lees AJ, Hardy J, Revesz T: Parkinson's disease. Lancet 2009;373:2055–2066.

14 Hughes AJ, Daniel SE, Kilford L, Lees AJ: Accuracy of clinical diagnosis of idiopathic Parkinson's disease: a clinicopathological study of 100 cases. J Neurol Neurosurg Psychiatry 1992;55:181–184.

15 Rascol O, Goetz C, Koller W, Poewe W, Sampaio C: Treatment interventions for Parkinson's disease: an evidence based assessment. Lancet 2002;359:1589–1598.

16 Marras C, McDermott MP, Rochon PA, et al: Survival in Parkinson disease: thirteen-year follow-up of the DATATOP cohort. Neurology 2005;64:87–93.

17 Katzenschlager R, Head J, Schrag A, Ben-Shlomo Y, Evans A, Lees AJ; Parkinson's Disease Research Group of the United Kingdom: Fourteen-year final report of the randomized PDRG-UK trial comparing three initial treatments in PD. Neurology 2008;71:474–480.

18 EMA/CHMP/330418/2012 rev 2. www. ema.europa.eu/.../WC500129601.pdf.

19 Martínez-Martín P, Gil-Nagel A, Gracia LM, Gómez JB, Martínez-Sarriés J, Bermejo F: Unified Parkinson's Disease Rating Scale characteristics and structure. The Cooperative Multicentric Group. Mov Disord 1994;9:76–83.

20 Vogt T, Kramer K, Gartenschlaeger M, Schreckenberger M: Estimation of further disease progression of Parkinson's disease by dopamin transporter scan vs. clinical rating. Parkinsonism Relat Disord 2011;17:459–463.

21 Gallagher CL, Johnson SC, Bendlin BB, et al: A longitudinal study of motor performance and striatal [^{18}F]fluorodopa uptake in Parkinson's disease. Brain Imaging Behav 2011;5:203–211.

22 Diener HC, Solbach K, Holle D, Gaul C: Integrated care for chronic migraine patients: epidemiology, burden, diagnosis and treatment options. Clin Med 2015;15:344–350.

23 Lanteri-Minet M: Economic burden and costs of chronic migraine. Curr Pain Headache Rep 2014;18:385.

24 Lenaerts ME: Burden of tension-type headache. Curr Pain Headache Rep 2006;10:459–462.

25 Becker WJ: Acute migraine treatment in adults. Headache 2015;55:778–793.

26 Millea PJ, Brodie JJ: Tension-type headache. Am Fam Physician 2002;66:797–804.

27 Weatherall MW: Drug therapy in headache. Clin Med 2015;15:273–279.

28 Headache Classification Committee of the International Headache Society: The International Classification of Headache Disorders, 3rd edition (beta version). Cephalalgia 2013;33:629–808.

29 Silberstein SD: Headaches in pregnancy. Neurol Clin 2004;22:727–756.

30 Forsgren L, Beghi E, Oun A, Sillanpää M: The epidemiology of epilepsy in Europe – a systematic review. Eur J Neurol 2005;12:245–253.

31 Sander JW: The epidemiology of epilepsy revisited. Curr Opin Neurol 2003;16: 165–170.

32 Fisher RS, Acevedo C, Arzimanoglou A, et al: ILAE official report: a practical clinical definition of epilepsy. Epilepsia 2014;55:475–482.

33 Annegers JF, Rocca WA, Hauser WA: Causes of epilepsy: contributions of the Rochester Epidemiology Project. Mayo Clin Proc 1996;71:570–575.

34 Shorvon SD, Goodridge DM: Longitudinal cohort studies of the prognosis of epilepsy: contribution of the National General Practice Study of Epilepsy and other studies. Brain 2013;136:3497–3510.

35 Sillanpää M, Schmidt D: Natural history of treated childhood-onset epilepsy: prospective, long-term population-based study. Brain 2006;129:617–624.

36 Nabbout R, Dulac O: Epileptic syndromes in infancy and childhood. Curr Opin Neurol 2008;21:161–166.

37 Beghi E, Carpio A, Forsgren L, et al: Recommendation for a definition of acute symptomatic seizure. Epilepsia 2010;51: 671–675.

38 Houtchens MK, Lublin FD, Miller AE, Khoury SJ: Multiple sclerosis and other inflammatory demyelinating diseases of the central nervous system; in: Daroff RB, Fenichel GM, Jankovic J, Mazziotta JC (eds): Bradley's Neurology in Clinical Practice, ed 6. Philadelphia, Saunders Elsevier, 2012.

39 Polman CH, Reingold SC, Banwell B, et al: Diagnostic criteria for multiple sclerosis: 2010 revisions to the McDonald criteria. Ann Neurol 2011;69:292–302.

40 Ascherio A: Environmental factors in multiple sclerosis. Expert Rev Neurother 2013;13(suppl 12):3–9.

41 Scalfari A, Neuhaus A, Degenhardt A, et al: The natural history of multiple sclerosis: a geographically based study 10: relapses and long-term disability. Brain 2010;133:1914–1929.

42 Lublin FD, Reingold SC, Cohen JA, et al: Defining the clinical course of multiple sclerosis: the 2013 revisions. Neurology 2014;83:278–286.

43 Miller D, Barkhof F, Montalban X, Thompson A, Filippi M: Clinically isolated syndromes suggestive of multiple sclerosis. Part I: natural history, pathogenesis, diagnosis, and prognosis. Lancet Neurol 2005;4:281–288.

44 Thrower BW: Relapse management in multiple sclerosis. Neurologist 2009;15: 1–5.

45 Sedal L, Wilson IB, McDonald EA: Current management of relapsing-remitting multiple sclerosis. Intern Med J 2014;44: 950–957.

46 Tanasescu R, Ionete C, Chou IJ, Constantinescu CS: Advances in the treatment of relapsing-remitting multiple sclerosis. Biomed J 2014;37:41–49.

47 Polman CH, O'Connor PW, Havrdova E, et al: A randomized, placebo-controlled trial of natalizumab for relapsing multiple sclerosis. N Engl J Med 2006;354: 899–910.

48 Kappos L, Radue EW, O'Connor P, et al: A placebo-controlled trial of oral fingolimod in relapsing multiple sclerosis. N Engl J Med 2010;362:387–401.

49 EMA/CHMP/771815/2011, Rev 2. www.ema.europa.eu/.../WC500133438.pdf.

50 Kurtzke JF: Rating neurologic impairment in multiple sclerosis: an expanded disability status scale (EDSS). Neurology 1983;33:1444–1452.

51 Rowland LP, Shneider NA: Amyotrophic lateral sclerosis. N Engl J Med 2001;344:1688–1700.

52 Tiryaki E, Horak HA: ALS and other motor neuron diseases. Continuum (Minneap Minn) 2014;20:1185–1207.

53 Ingre C, Roos PM, Piehl F, Kamel F, Fang F: Risk factors for amyotrophic lateral sclerosis. Clin Epidemiol 2015;7:181–193.

54 Swinnen B, Robberecht W: The phenotypic variability of amyotrophic lateral sclerosis. Nat Rev Neurol 2014;10:661–670.

55 Pupillo E, Messina P, Logroscino G, Beghi E; SLALOM Group: Long-term survival in amyotrophic lateral sclerosis: a population-based study. Ann Neurol 2014;75:287–297.

56 Miller RG, Mitchell JD, Moore DH: Riluzole for amyotrophic lateral sclerosis (ALS)/motor neuron disease (MND). Cochrane Database Syst Rev 2012;3:CD001447.

57 Chiò A, Logroscino G, Traynor BJ, et al: Global epidemiology of amyotrophic lateral sclerosis: a systematic review of the published literature. Neuroepidemiology 2013;41:118–130.

58 Cedarbaum JM, Stambler N, Malta E, et al: The ALSFRS-R: a revised ALS functional rating scale that incorporates assessments of respiratory function. BDNF ALS Study Group (Phase III). J Neurol Sci 1999;169:13–21.

59 Castrillo-Viguera C, Grasso DL, Simpson E, Shefner J, Cudkowicz ME: Clinical significance in the change of decline in ALSFRS-R. Amyotroph Lateral Scler 2010;11:178–180.

60 Medical Research Council: Aids to the Investigation of Peripheral Nerve Injuries. War Memorandum, ed 2. London, HMSO, 1943, vol 7, pp 11–46.

61 EMA/CHMP/40105/2013. www.ema.europa.eu/.../WC500147005.pdf.

62 GBD 2013 Mortality and Causes of Death Collaborators: Global, regional, and national age-sex specific all-cause and cause-specific mortality for 240 causes of death, 1990–2013: a systematic analysis for the Global Burden of Disease Study 2013. Lancet 2015;385:117–171.

63 GBD 2013 DALYs and HALE Collaborators, Murray CJ, Barber RM, Foreman KJ, et al: Global, regional, and national disability-adjusted life years (DALYs) for 306 diseases and injuries and healthy life expectancy (HALE) for 188 countries, 1990–2013: quantifying the epidemiological transition. Lancet 2015;386:2145–2191.

64 Prabhakaran S, Ruff I, Bernstein RA: Acute stroke intervention: a systematic review. JAMA 2015;313:1451–1462.

65 Hong KS, Yegiaian S, Lee M, Lee J, Saver JL: Declining stroke and vascular event recurrence rates in secondary prevention trials over the past 50 years and consequences for current trial design. Circulation 2011;123:2111–2119.

66 Lyden PD, Lu M, Jackson C, Marler J, et al: Underlying structure of the National Institutes of Health Stroke Scale: results of a factor analysis. Stroke 1999;30:2347–2354.

67 Scandinavian Stroke Study Group: Multicenter trial of hemodilution in ischemic stroke – background and study protocol. Stroke 1985;16:885–890.

68 Stavem K, Lossius M, Rønning OM: Reliability and validity of the Canadian Neurological Scale in retrospective assessment of initial stroke severity. Cerebrovasc Dis 2003;16:286–291.

69 Edwards DF, Chen YW, Diringer MN: Unified Neurological Stroke Scale is valid in ischemic and hemorrhagic stroke. Stroke 1995;26:1852–1858.

70 Mahoney FI, Barthel D: Functional evaluation: the Barthel Index. Md State Med J 1965;14:56–61.

71 Banks JL, Marotta CA: Outcomes validity and reliability of the modified Rankin scale: implications for stroke clinical trials: a literature review and synthesis. Stroke 2007;38:1091–1096.

72 Jennett B, Bond M: Assessment of outcome after severe brain damage. A practical scale. Lancet 1975;1:480–484.

Ettore Beghi, MD
Laboratory of Neurological Disorders, IRCCS-Mario Negri
Institute for Pharmacological Research, Via Giuseppe La Masa 19
IT–20156 Milan (Italy)
E-Mail ettore.beghi@marionegri.it

Beghi E, Logroscino G (eds): The Right Therapy for Neurological Disorders. From Randomized Trials to Clinical Practice.
Front Neurol Neurosci. Basel, Karger, 2016, vol 39, pp 24–36 (DOI: 10.1159/000445410)

Current Issues in Randomized Clinical Trials of Neurodegenerative Disorders at Enrolment and Reporting: Diagnosis, Recruitment, Representativeness of Patients, Ethnicity, and Quality of Reporting

Giancarlo Logroscino[a, b] · Rosa Capozzo[a, b] · Rosanna Tortelli[a, b] · Benoît Marin[a–e]

[a]Department of Basic Medical Sciences, Neuroscience and Sense Organs, University of Bari 'Aldo Moro', Bari, and [b]Unit of Neurodegenerative Diseases, Department of Clinical Research in Neurology, University of Bari 'Aldo Moro', 'Pia Fondazione Cardinale G. Panico', Tricase, Italy; [c]INSERM, U1094, Tropical Neuroepidemiology, [d]UMR_S 1094, Tropical Neuroepidemiology, Institute of Neuroepidemiology and Tropical Neurology, CNRS FR 3503 GEIST, University of Limoges, and [e]Centre d'Epidémiologie de Biostatistique et de Méthodologie de la Recherche, CHU Limoges, Limoges, France

Abstract

Background: The investigator is faced with several challenges when planning a randomized clinical trial (RCT). In the early phase, issues are particularly challenging for RCTs in neurodegenerative disorders (NDD). ***Summary:*** At the time of inclusion in the study, an early and accurate diagnosis is mandatory. Variability of diagnostic criteria, mostly based on clinical grounds, lag time between onset and enrolment, and phenotypic heterogeneity are the main drivers of diagnostic complexity. High-quality data in terms of diagnostic reliability, phenotypic description, follow-up, and evaluation of outcomes are key determinants and are highly conditioned by the expertise of the investigators and center recruitment rate. Representativeness of NDD patients is mandatory to postulate the generalizability of the results of RCTs. There is, however, a systematic selection bias in terms of age (more likely to be younger), sex (more likely to be male), ethnicity (more likely to be of European/Caucasian origin), and other prognostic factors (more likely to be favorable). In the publication phase, researchers need to report properly all of the main features of the RCT. Consolidated Standards of Reporting Trials (CONSORT) facilitates the report and interpretation of RCTs, but adherence to these guidelines needs to be improved. ***Key Messages:*** Several issues discussed in this review may alter the internal and external validity of an RCT. To date, the impact on phenotype at study entry has often been overlooked. A differential effect of the selection of subjects and of specific clinical and nonclinical features needs to be systematically explored in the RCT planning phase. © 2016 S. Karger AG, Basel

There are several challenges at the beginning of a clinical trial that the investigator has to face – this chapter will be a quick survey of some of the more challenging issues connected to the inclusion of patients suffering from neurodegenerative disorders (NDDs) in a randomized clinical trial (RCT): the diagnosis, the selection process and related issues, and adherence to the Consolidated Standards of Reporting Trials (CONSORT) guidelines.

Diagnosis in Randomized Clinical Trials

The challenge of diagnosis in RCTs is similar for difficulties and ambiguities to what happens in the realm of everyday clinical practice. The correctness of the diagnosis of a specific clinical condition is what drives the enrolment in clinical trials. Several issues make the diagnosis of a neurological disorder particularly challenging especially in chronic diseases like NDDs. We are going to present the case of NDDs as a possible example of issues present in the inception of patients to be enrolled in an RCT.

The main issues related to diagnosis are the following: (1) the diagnostic criteria are extremely variable and based mainly on clinical grounds, (2) the diagnostic criteria have recently been changing and now include advanced technology like imaging or fluid biomarkers from plasma and cerebrospinal fluid, (3) the time interval between disease onset at the pathological level and first clinical symptom can be extremely heterogeneous and of exceptional duration, probably measurable even in decades, (4) the clinical presentation and course of different diseases may be different by age group, sex, and ethnicity.

In the last years, one of the focuses of clinical research in neurodegenerative diseases has been the need to anticipate the clinical diagnosis with the utilization of imaging and fluid biomarkers. This approach has been largely used in Alzheimer's disease (AD) and it is beginning to be used or proposed in Parkinson's disease (PD) and amyotrophic lateral sclerosis (ALS). This is key to implementing future RCTs. This approach is still in the early phase and all the implications of this approach are not entirely clear.

The Early Diagnosis Problem: The Example of Parkinson's Disease

There is a clear conflict between the need to have an early diagnosis and the certainty of the diagnosis. Early diagnosis is needed to have more chances to detect an efficacious treatment, in both symptomatic and disease-modifying treatment. A considerable amount of cells is dead in significant areas of the brain when clinical diagnosis is finally obtained. The certainty of the diagnosis is important because the introduction of a false-positive diagnosis would decrease the power of any study, including an RCT. We can use the example of PD. The two main sets of clinical criteria used for the diagnosis are the UK Brain Bank (UKBB) criteria [1] and the National Institute of Neurological and Stroke Disorders (NINDS) criteria, also known as the Gelb criteria [2]. In both there is one set of three cardinal criteria: bradykinesia, resting tremor, and rigidity. The fourth is postural instability in the UKBB and unilateral onset in the NINDS criteria. The NINDS criteria also add a set of exclusion criteria to identify non-PD parkinsonism. The timing of onset of other clinical features after the first motor symptom is critical: postural instability, hallucinations, and freezing phenomena in the first 3 years, and dementia preceding motor symptoms or occurring within the first year are suggestive of alternative diagnoses. In a trial of PD, the inclusion of subjects with progressive supranuclear palsy, corticobasal degeneration, and multisystem atrophy would endanger the results of the study. All these phenotypes have a negative prognosis and are poorly responsive to therapies for PD. On the other hand, the inclusion of subjects with essential tremor, wrongly diagnosed as PD, would falsely shift the overall estimate of prognosis towards a better prognosis.

One of the main problems is that all current diagnostic criteria include lists of signs and symptoms for inclusion as well as for exclusion criteria in the early stages of disease. This is clearly stated in the NINDS criteria where we need at least 3 years to have a sufficient time lag to look for specific inclusion and exclusion symptoms and signs. The diagnosis therefore can be changed in some patients with parkinsonism after a clinical follow-up of a few years [3]. Symptom duration of at least 3 years is necessary to meet the requirement for a diagnosis of probable PD, the highest degree of diagnostic certainty without pathological confirmation. In a recent meta-analysis on diagnostic accuracy, the positive predictive value of nonexperts increased from around 75–85% after few years after the first visit [4]. Time to first symptom is probably the main issue, with a positive predictive value that reached 53% in patients with <5 years of disease duration and even 26% in patients with <3 years of disease duration in one study [5]. This can be a major problem for RCTs if they are designed to recruit patients at the beginning of the natural history of PD [6], when the possible positive effects of a drug are more likely.

Movement disorder experts are generally involved in the recruitment and follow-up of patients for RCTs in tertiary referral centers and are often indicated as the gold standard in validity studies on PD diagnostic criteria. Movement disorder experts, however, improve the quality of diagnosis only slightly. The improvement of positive predictive value in series where the diagnosis is made by a movement disorder expert was less than 10% (as compared to less experienced professionals) when their diagnostic accuracy was tested against the pathological examination as the gold standard.

Interestingly, the accuracy of PD diagnosis did not improve in the last 25 years [4]. In a disease where there have been no major changes in classification criteria and diagnostic procedures, the number of subjects with a correct diagnosis is far from optimal: 8 out of 10.

This example shows that we need some years to increase the validity of the diagnosis, but this happens in a phase where the neuropathological damage is already substantial. This statement can be broadly applied to all neurodegenerative diseases.

Selection for Randomized Clinical Trials: The Role of Recruitment Site

A major source of patient selection in a clinical trial is the center where the trial is conducted. The recent guidelines named SPIRIT report that the countries, type of setting, and number of sites of trial should be clearly described because these RCT features have important effects on recruitment success, attrition, and outcomes. Therefore, the characteristics of study sites determine both internal and external validity [7]. The proper selection and enrolment of patients for RCTs in neurological disorders depend on the expertise and the training levels of the different researchers. In centers with experience in the diagnosis, reliable diagnostic criteria, and selection methods are applied, but this may not be the same for centers with relatively less experience. Recently, with the rapid development of new therapies to be tested particularly in dementias, new clinical sites that lack high diagnostic experience are being involved in the recruitment of patients for research. While this increases the feasibility of sample size completeness, this also determines the variability in patient selection for clinical trials, which may not be consistent across sites in multicenter studies. Findings from a large multicenter RCT, aiming to evaluate the efficacy of estrogens to prevent AD, underlined the difficulties of conducting a study and managing data from sites that lack a high level of expertise in the neurological field. This study highlighted the importance of including an administrative and data-coordinating center at the main site responsible for data collection and monitoring. This is mandatory to minimize differences among sites [8]. As a result, we face another source of contrast between the need to enroll large numbers and the different quality of diagnosis in the sites of a multicenter RCT.

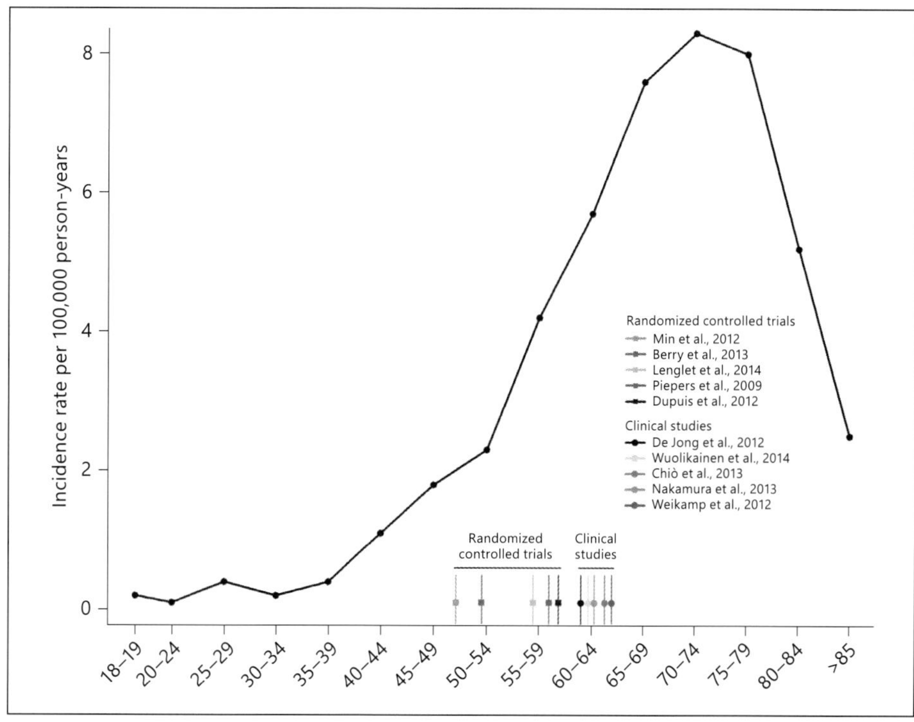

Fig. 1. Age-specific incidence rates of ALS in Europe over a 2-year period, 1998–1999 (adapted from Logroscino et al. [59]). Bars indicate the mean age of patients enrolled in each of the five RCTs (squares) [18–20, 23, 25] and five clinical studies (circles) [21, 22, 24, 26, 27] of ALS randomly selected as examples.

Selection for Randomized Clinical Trials: The Role of Age and Sex

More problems are due to selection processes that affect both the internal and external validity of RCTs. The priority given to the rapidity of patient enrolment may likely be responsible for the poor representativeness of subjects enrolled in clinical trials [9].

The exclusion of subjects belonging to the oldest age group is a common practice in RCTs in NDDs. In PD RCTs, the average age is 64 years [10–13]. The same problem is present in AD RCTs where the average age is 74 years [14–16]. This is in contrast with the epidemiological evidence showing that in these diseases the peak of incidence increases with age and is still increasing after age 90 (aging-related diseases). The alternative model (age-related diseases) displays a peak in the mid-70s or early 80s followed by a rapid decrease [17]. ALS studies suffer from similar problems: both RCTs and clinical studies generally tend to enroll patients in lower ages and this is particularly evident for RCTs [18–27] (fig. 1). This could be explained by the fact that older patients are less likely to be referred to a tertiary center of care and thus to be selected for research [28]. The debate of what is the more appropriate model is still open. We do not have evidence to prefer one model over another, but the aging model is probably more appropriate in AD, while the second model is more appropriate for PD and ALS. In both cases the peak of the age curve of the patients enrolled in a clinical trial is at a much lower age than in the source population of the participants of the RCT.

People aged ≥85 years, the oldest-old, represent the fastest growing slice of the population, accounting for about 12% of those aged >65 years [29]. With the increasing number of subjects in this age group, studies are needed to better analyze whether they present sociodemographic differences or different risk/protective factors compared to the younger-old, including response to treatment. Age of subjects in RCTs may also determine important influences on the response to therapies. For example, a study aiming to assess the response to the anticholinesterase inhibitor donepezil in 282 AD patients found improved cognitive functioning in over 65% of patients reaching 3 months (n = 184) and 51% on intention-to-treat analysis (n = 231), with significantly greater improvement (p = 0.03) in those aged 65 and under [30]. The best possible effect is probably restricted to a small group of potential candidates.

Nonetheless, in many studies there is an artificial upper limit that is applied [15, 31], reducing the applicability of the results of the study in this age group. This limit is posed for example in more than 60% of recent AD trials and in about 50% of PD clinical trials. This means the exclusion of more than 50% of potential candidates to study entry. In PD, exclusion by an arbitrary upper age limit is common and 79.3 years (range 64–95 years) is the mean upper age limit for exclusion of subjects from trials. Exclusion by age is primarily applied in smaller studies, in particular those with less than 100 subjects [32]. Therefore, the exclusion of older participants significantly limits the generalization of results obtained from PD research to the high amount of elderly PD patients seen in clinical practice [32].

In several studies [33–35] of early PD, the average age at entry is in the early 60s, quite different from real average age of onset of PD [36]. The disease duration from two Parkinson studies of patients in more advanced stages of disease is 9 years [37, 38], although the average age at the time of study entry is in the early 60s. Conversely, individuals with 10 years of PD are expected to be in their early 70s. This supports the hypothesis that subject samples recruited in clinical trials may not be fully representative of the real target population of subjects with the disease.

It is important to underline that there are several obstacles to the enrolment of elderly subjects in RCT. First, elderly subjects are less likely to fulfil eligibility criteria compared to younger subjects. Furthermore, the elderly are less likely to participate in research and especially to stay during the follow-up required in an RCT. Nonetheless, a recent study reported that AD prevention trials can enroll elderly participants with a minimal impact on trial retention and that enriching for older individuals (limiting trial populations to those at least age 70 or 75 years) reduces the number of participants needed to adequately power a trial [39]. Relative to the standard trial model enrolling participants aged 65 years or older, trials with a minimum age requirement of 70 and 75 years reduce the necessary trial sample sizes by 8 and 18%, respectively. Contrary to their first hypothesis, the authors neither observed an increase in the dropout rate nor a reduction in the eligibility rate in the older populations [39] (fig. 2).

Similar problems have been described in ALS. Patients enrolled in ALS clinical trials are demographically and clinically different from the ALS cohorts based on recruitment in population-based settings. Factors such as younger age, spinal onset, male gender, and regular attendance at an ALS center strongly increase the chance of being enrolled in a clinical trial. All these characteristics are favorable prognostic factors [40]. The different survivorship in an observational setting between patients with these characteristics has been estimated to be 1 year, more than half of the median survivorship of an ALS patient according to EURALS data [40]. The subjects selected for trials are more likely to have a longer survivorship and this may at least partially explain the negative results of ALS trials [9]. Age and other

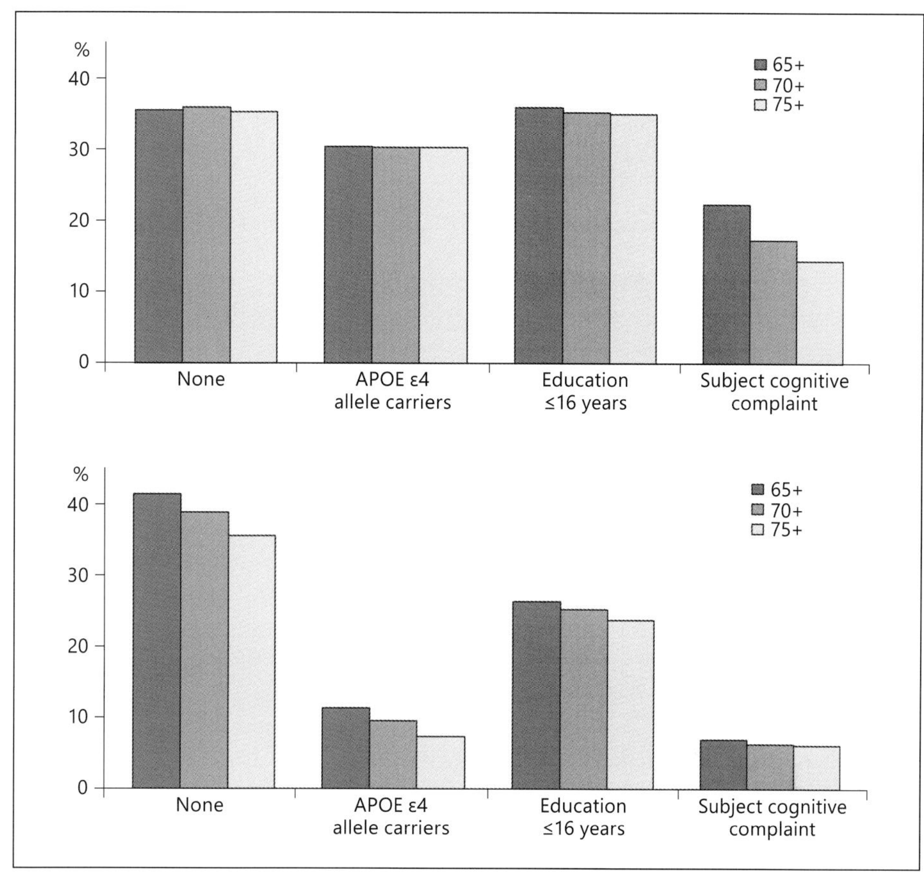

Fig. 2. The impact of age on eligibility and dropout rate (%) at 3 years for varying enrichment strategies in the Alzheimer's Disease Prevention Trial. Adapted from Grill and Monsell [39].

characteristics also limit the external validity of the results' representativeness of subjects enrolled in an RCT and the possibility to extend their results to the whole ALS population [9] (fig. 3).

Sex is a key variable in subgroup analysis of RCTs, particularly for those conforming with international quality standards and primarily for AD RCT [14, 31, 41]. AD affects more women than men with a male-female incidence ratio between 1.2 and 1.5. Several pieces of evidence report sex differences in the clinical picture, living conditions, and response to therapies, which may affect outcomes in clinical trials in patients with AD. Therefore, the inadequate consideration of this variable may determine a selection bias, thus reducing the applicability of the results of clinical trials to the general population [42].

Recent evidence shows that only 62% of RCTs on psychosocial outcomes in AD and mild cognitive impairment report the sex ratio, and women are significantly underrepresented in studies reporting this ratio [31]. Furthermore, only a third of the studies reporting sex distribution also report analysis of sex effects on treatment outcomes. The underrepresentation of females may be due to a bias in sampling. In many AD trials, the availability of the caregiver present during the entire study period is an inclusion criterion. Because of the demographic structure of the oldest age groups with a longer survivorship of females,

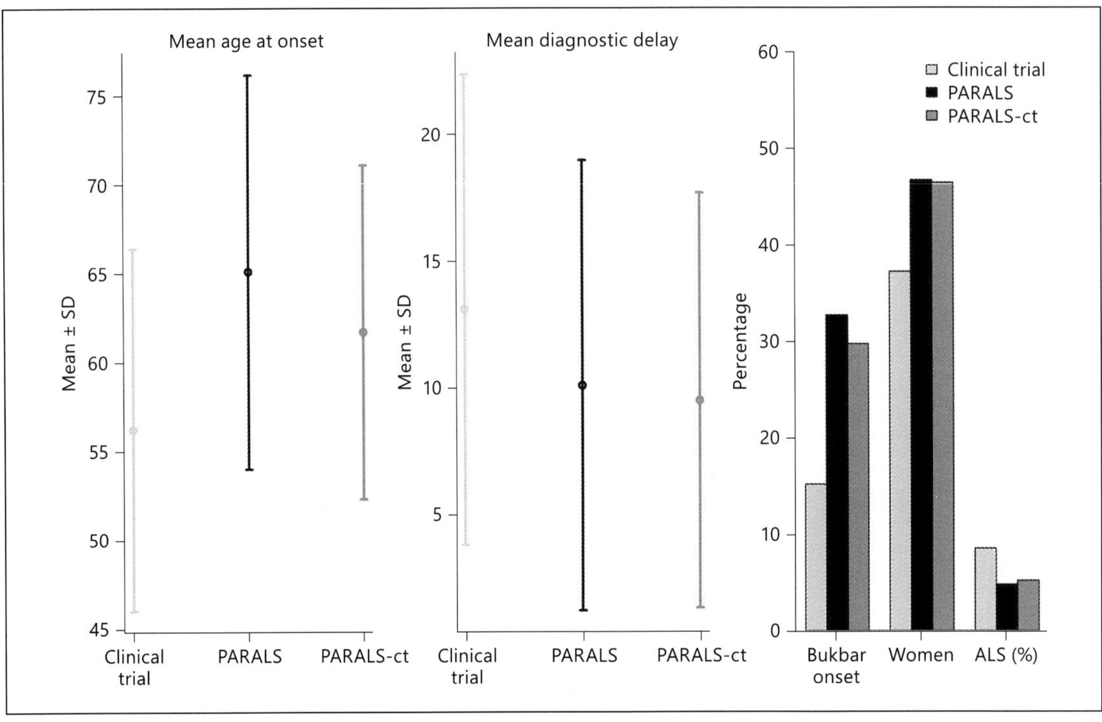

Fig. 3. Comparison of characteristics of patients enrolled in 8 clinical trials run by Turin ALS center, in PARALS (Piemonte and Valle d'Aosta register of ALS), and in PARALS-ct (PARALS patients meeting the usual criteria for inclusion in clinical trials). Adapted from Chiò et al. [9].

the caregivers of AD patients are mostly women/spouses, which likely contributes to the male predominance [43].

Selection for Randomized Clinical Trials: The Role of Ethnicity

Ethnicity in RCTs is a factor of importance because there are elements to support differences between human populations in the clinical expression of NDDs at the time of diagnosis, during the course, and in outcomes [44, 45]. This has been postulated thanks to descriptions of ALS, PD, and AD phenotype from various populations [46–49], reviews and meta-analyses [50–53], and studies performed in multiethnic countries such as the US or the UK [54–56]. For example, young-

onset cases of NDDs might be more frequent in African populations as compared to Europeans [46, 57, 58]. The sex ratio appears different among populations: close to 1 for ALS in populations of European origin versus >1 in other populations [50, 51], and close to 1 for PD in Asia versus >1 in European populations [52]. Disease-specific differences between ethnic groups have also been described: (1) more frequent bulbar-onset ALS in Northern Europe as compared to other European populations [59], (2) more frequent personality and functional changes associated with AD before signs of cognitive impairment in African-Americans as compared to Whites [55] and more dementia-related behaviors, along with Hispanics [55, 56]. Poorer outcomes, including survival, have been documented for ALS and AD in ethnic minorities in the US and in the UK [55, 60], while

PD progression could be slower in 25% of African cases as compared to European patients [61]. Differences could be related to differences in efficiency and access to health systems.

Differences in treatment outcome, drug metabolism, and adverse events are highly probable but, to date, are impossible to fully investigate [62]. It is also impossible to decipher if variation with ethnicity would mainly be driven by the population's ancestral origin, other genetic factors (uneven distribution of high-risk or protective genes) [63, 64], population demographic characteristics, or environmental, social, or cultural factors [54, 65].

Ethnicity is, up to now, insufficiently considered in design or analysis of RCTs in NDD. By searching for the most recent RCTs published in highly impacted journals and with the highest number of citations (up to five articles by disease), we found that no RCT on ALS [18, 23, 66] or PD [10–13, 67] mentioned the ancestral origin or ethnicity of recruited patients. The situation was different for AD. Out of five publications, one did not report the ethnicity of included patients [14] while four did. In two of those, 95% of the subjects were White subjects [15, 31], whereas only two RCTs included multiethnic patients: Whites for a majority of cases (65–85%), but also Asians, African-Americans, and Hispanics/Latinos, with variation in those distributions depending on the sites of recruitment [16, 68]. Ethnicity distribution was displayed for comparability assessment between groups, but no subgroup analysis was performed to identify any interaction between treatment effect and ethnicity. The overall picture illustrates that some ethnic groups are poorly represented in worldwide RCTs, as is the case in biomarker studies [62]. The differential access to health care experienced by developing countries and ethnic minorities in Western countries might be a reason for the reduced access to trials testing new drugs. As compared to Whites, African-Americans and Hispanics with dementia or ALS have a lower or delayed access to diagnostic services and experience less accurate diagnosis [55, 69–71]. This referral issue, along with inadequate treatment, determines outcomes [55]. Barriers to help-seeking and in the diagnosis pathway are related to economic problems (poverty, lower access to health insurance or specialist care, excluding patients from identified as eligible for research), culture (beliefs about the cause, concerns about stigma, ethical imperative to care for one's own family), and social factors (negative experience with health system, language barriers) [54, 72, 73].

The Issue of Sample Representativeness in Randomized Clinical Trials: The Example of Alzheimer's Disease

Advancing research and clinical care and conducting cost-effective and successful RCTs require the proper characterization of a given patient population. Subject selection and exclusion criteria employed in a typical efficacy RCT of investigational new drugs is based on two principal aims: (1) to identify patients truly suffering from the condition the drug is intended to treat, and (2) to maximize the probability that the study will detect an effect of the drug, if it exists.

The extensive clinical heterogeneity of patients with NDDs is a great concern in designing clinical trials. AD represents the best example of a complex disease with an heterogeneous clinical and pathological expression likely contributing to treatment response variability among patients. Medical comorbidities may further complicate the clinical picture or affect outcome. This issue concerns especially the study of AD and related dementias, which are predominantly conditions of older subjects carrying a high number of comorbid diseases. Sponsors of RCTs try to overcome this issue by using restrictive selection criteria for subjects enrolled in trials, mainly on the basis of age and comorbidity [74].

Accordingly, few patients may be qualified to participate in RCTs. The dementia population enrolled in these trials generally consists of mildly to moderately impaired outpatients living at home with caregivers, with a diagnosis of probable AD using the NINCDS-ADRDA workshop criteria [75]. Study subjects are further required to be healthy, without significant medical illness and psychiatric disorders, and with normal blood screening tests. Additional inclusion and exclusion criteria of RCTs vary with respect to each different medication to test. In clinical trials, AD patients are generally recruited from memory clinics, hospitals, and nursing homes, thus creating a selection bias [76].

A recent study analyzing the selection of AD patients in RCTs reported that the most frequent reasons for not including some patients in AD trials are abnormalities on MRI (56%, of which 89% are white matter lesions), unauthorized drugs (37%), the absence of a study partner/informant (37%), comorbidities (25%), visual/auditory impairments (3%), alcohol abuse (2%), and inadequate educational level (1%) [77]. Nonetheless, many observational epidemiological studies have highlighted the frequent association between cerebrovascular pathology and AD; vascular risk factors are also reported as risk factors for AD [78, 79].

Both the stringency of selection criteria and the variability among trials may be responsible for the enrolment of subgroups of patients who are not representative of the AD population in clinical practice. Therefore, disqualifying many potential subjects from participation in clinical trials could limit the external validity of trial results.

Randomized Clinical Trials: Compliance with CONSORT Guidelines

'The whole of medicine depends on the transparent reporting of clinical trials' [80]. Well-designed and properly conducted RCTs provide the most reliable evidence on the efficacy of health care interventions, while trials with inadequate methods are greatly associated with bias, in particular when a positive effect of treatment is reported [81]. Misleading decision-making in health care at all levels, from therapy decisions for a patient to formulation of national public health policies, may be generated by biased results derived from poorly designed and reported trials.

A group of scientists and editors developed the CONSORT statement to improve the quality of reporting in RCTs. CONSORT was first published in 1996 [82], updated in 2001 [80], and revised in 2010 [83]. CONSORT consists of a checklist and flowchart that authors can use for reporting results from an RCT. The statement facilitates critical appraisal and interpretation of RCTs. Accordingly, several leading medical journals and major international editorial groups have endorsed the CONSORT statement. Nonetheless, a recent study examining the content of 35 journals' instructions to authors, reported that only 4% of all words were addressed to the content of the abstract format. Journal instructions provide little guidance about methodological and statistical issues, and the material provided is often contradictory among journals [84].

Clear, transparent, and sufficiently detailed abstracts related to RCTs are important because readers often base their initial evaluation of a trial on the information reported in the abstract, in particular when the full publication is not available. Currently, the CONSORT statement recommends what information should be reported in the abstract describing an RCT.

Considering that many reviews have documented deficiencies in clinical trials with adherence to CONSORT guidelines [85, 86], we decided, as an example, to evaluate the level of adherence of RCTs indexed in PubMed in 2014 and 2015 regarding four neurodegenerative diseases: AD, PD, ALS, and frontotemporal dementia. We restricted the evaluation to the CONSORT guidelines for abstracts. They are structured in 16 items: title, trial design, six items for the methods section (participants, interventions, objective, outcome, randomization, blinding), five items for

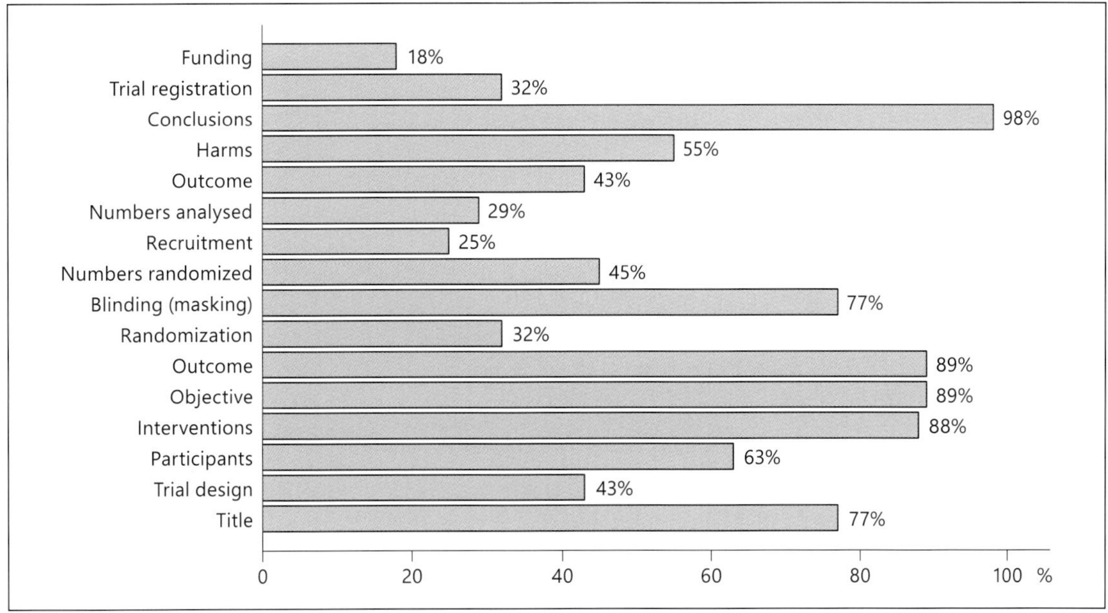

Fig. 4. Percentage of compliance to the list of items of CONSORT in a sample of recent RCTs in neurodegenerative diseases.

results section (numbers randomized, recruitment, numbers analyzed, outcome, harms), conclusions, trial registration, and funding. We identified 54 RCTs from January 2014 to April 2015 (28 for AD, 20 for PD, and 5 for ALS). Furthermore, we did not consider temporal limits for frontotemporal dementia because of the lack of RCTs; we found and considered 3 RCTs for frontotemporal dementia, published in 2004, 2013, and 2015. We analyzed the abstracts of 57 RCTs in total. None of them followed 100% of the CONSORT guidelines: 15 studies (26%) adhered to >70% of items, 34 studies (60%) complied with 50–70% of the items, and 8 studies (14%) observed a number of items <50%. The most adhered to item (98% of cases) was 'conclusions'; the least adhered to item (18% of cases) was 'funding'. Figure 4 shows the percentage of adherence for each item of the considered RCTs. This review shows that, as in other topics, adherence of trial reports to CONSORT guidelines needs to be improved in the field of NDDs.

Conclusions

The diagnosis that is the first step for in inclusion in RCT is often delayed because of many factors. The entry of subjects in clinical trials should be limited to incident cases or cases with a short natural history. The early diagnosis is challenged by phenotype, older age, female sex, and comorbidities [74]. Biological characteristics play a major role, but we should not underestimate the importance of social factors affecting inclusion, such as access to specialized medical care, education, and social status.

There is a need for (1) a better consideration of key descriptive elements of the patients recruited (center, age, sex, ethnicity) and the representativeness of the sample, and (2) a better consideration of these issues (age, sex, ethnicity) in the results of the RCT (interaction with efficacy or side effects of treatment).

Most of the issues dealt with in this review have an effect on both internal and external validity of RCTs.

References

1 Hughes AJ, Daniel SE, Kilford L, et al: Accuracy of clinical diagnosis of idiopathic Parkinson's disease: a clinico-pathological study of 100 cases. J Neurol Neurosurg Psychiatry 1992;55:181–184.

2 Gelb DJ, Oliver E, Gilman S: Diagnostic criteria for Parkinson disease. Arch Neurol 1999;56:33–39.

3 Berg D, Lang AE, Postuma RB, et al: Changing the research criteria for the diagnosis of Parkinson's disease: obstacles and opportunities. Lancet Neurol 2013;12:514–524.

4 Rizzo G, Arcuti S, Martino D, et al: Accuracy of clinical diagnosis of Parkinson's disease: a systematic review and Bayesian meta-analysis. Neurology 2016;86:566–576.

5 Adler CH, Beach TG, Hentz JG, et al: Low clinical diagnostic accuracy of early vs advanced Parkinson disease: clinico-pathologic study. Neurology 2014;83:406–412.

6 Poewe W: The natural history of Parkinson's disease. J Neurol 2006;253(suppl 7):VII2–VII6.

7 Chan AW, Tetzlaff JM, Gotzsche PC, et al: SPIRIT 2013 explanation and elaboration: guidance for protocols of clinical trials. BMJ 2013;346:e7586.

8 Sano M, Jacobs D, Andrews H, et al: A multi-center, randomized, double blind placebo-controlled trial of estrogens to prevent Alzheimer's disease and loss of memory in women: design and baseline characteristics. Clin Trials 2008;5:523–533.

9 Chio A, Canosa A, Gallo S, et al: ALS clinical trials: do enrolled patients accurately represent the ALS population? Neurology 2011;77:1432–1437.

10 Lewitt PA, Hauser RA, Lu M, et al: Randomized clinical trial of fipamezole for dyskinesia in Parkinson disease (FJORD study). Neurology 2012;79:163–169.

11 Lewitt PA, Guttman M, Tetrud JW, et al: Adenosine A2A receptor antagonist istradefylline (KW-6002) reduces 'off' time in Parkinson's disease: a double-blind, randomized, multicenter clinical trial (6002-US-005). Ann Neurol 2008;63:295–302.

12 Espay AJ, Dwivedi AK, Payne M, et al: Methylphenidate for gait impairment in Parkinson disease: a randomized clinical trial. Neurology 2011;76:1256–1262.

13 Parkinson Study Group QEI, Beal MF, Oakes D, et al: A randomized clinical trial of high-dosage coenzyme Q10 in early Parkinson disease: no evidence of benefit. JAMA Neurol 2014;71:543–552.

14 Geldmacher DS, Fritsch T, Mcclendon MJ, et al: A randomized pilot clinical trial of the safety of pioglitazone in treatment of patients with Alzheimer disease. Arch Neurol 2011;68:45–50.

15 Dodel R, Rominger A, Bartenstein P, et al: Intravenous immunoglobulin for treatment of mild-to-moderate Alzheimer's disease: a phase 2, randomised, double-blind, placebo-controlled, dose-finding trial. Lancet Neurol 2013;12:233–243.

16 Porsteinsson AP, Drye LT, Pollock BG, et al: Effect of citalopram on agitation in Alzheimer disease: the CitAD randomized clinical trial. JAMA 2014;311:682–691.

17 Logroscino G, Tortelli R, Rizzo G, et al. Amyotrophic lateral sclerosis: an aging-related disease. Curr Geri Rep 2015;4:142–153.

18 Dupuis L, Dengler R, Heneka MT, et al: A randomized, double blind, placebo-controlled trial of pioglitazone in combination with riluzole in amyotrophic lateral sclerosis. PLoS One 2012;7:e37885.

19 Min JH, Hong YH, Sung JJ, et al: Oral solubilized ursodeoxycholic acid therapy in amyotrophic lateral sclerosis: a randomized cross-over trial. J Korean Med Sci 2012;27:200–206.

20 Berry JD, Shefner JM, Conwit R, et al: Design and initial results of a multiphase randomized trial of ceftriaxone in amyotrophic lateral sclerosis. PLoS One 2013;8:e61177.

21 Chio A, Mora G, Restagno G, et al: UNC13A influences survival in Italian amyotrophic lateral sclerosis patients: a population-based study. Neurobiol Aging 2013;34:357.e1–e5.

22 De Jong SW, Huisman MH, Sutedja NA, et al: Smoking, alcohol consumption, and the risk of amyotrophic lateral sclerosis: a population-based study. Am J Epidemiol 2012;176:233–239.

23 Lenglet T, Lacomblez L, Abitbol JL, et al: A phase II–III trial of olesoxime in subjects with amyotrophic lateral sclerosis. Eur J Neurol 2014;21:529–536.

24 Nakamura R, Atsuta N, Watanabe H, et al: Neck weakness is a potent prognostic factor in sporadic amyotrophic lateral sclerosis patients. J Neurol Neurosurg Psychiatry 2013;84:1365–1371.

25 Piepers S, Veldink JH, De Jong SW, et al: Randomized sequential trial of valproic acid in amyotrophic lateral sclerosis. Ann Neurol 2009;66:227–234.

26 Wuolikainen A, Acimovic J, Lovgren-Sandblom A, et al: Cholesterol, oxysterol, triglyceride, and coenzyme Q homeostasis in ALS. Evidence against the hypothesis that elevated 27-hydroxycholesterol is a pathogenic factor. PLoS One 2014;9:e113619.

27 Weikamp JG, Schelhaas HJ, Hendriks JC, et al: Prognostic value of decreased tongue strength on survival time in patients with amyotrophic lateral sclerosis. J Neurol 2012;259:2360–2365.

28 Logroscino G, Traynor BJ, Hardiman O, et al: Descriptive epidemiology of amyotrophic lateral sclerosis: new evidence and unsolved issues. J Neurol Neurosurg Psychiatry 2008;79:6–11.

29 Kawas CH: The oldest old and the 90+ Study. Alzheimers Dement 2008;4:S56–S59.

30 Evans M, Ellis A, Watson D, et al: Sustained cognitive improvement following treatment of Alzheimer's disease with donepezil. Int J Geriatr Psychiatry 2000;15:50–53.

31 Salloway S, Sperling R, Fox NC, et al: Two phase 3 trials of bapineuzumab in mild-to-moderate Alzheimer's disease. N Engl J Med 2014;370:322–333.

32 Fitzsimmons PR, Blayney S, Mina-Corkill S, et al: Older participants are frequently excluded from Parkinson's disease research. Parkinsonism Relat Disord 2012;18:585–589.

33 Parkinson Study Group: Effects of tocopherol and deprenyl on the progression of disability in early Parkinson's disease. N Engl J Med 1993;328:176–183.

34 Fahn S, Oakes D, Shoulson I, et al: Levodopa and the progression of Parkinson's disease. N Engl J Med 2004;351:2498–2508.

35 Parkinson Study Group: A controlled, randomized, delayed-start study of rasagiline in early Parkinson disease. Arch Neurol 2004;61:561–566.

36 Wang V, Chao TH, Hsieh CC, et al: Cancer risks among the users of ergot-derived dopamine agonists for Parkinson's disease, a nationwide population-based survey. Parkinsonism Relat Disord 2015; 21:18–22.

37 Parkinson Study Group: A randomized placebo-controlled trial of rasagiline in levodopa-treated patients with Parkinson disease and motor fluctuations: the PRESTO study. Arch Neurol 2005;62: 241–248.

38 Entacapone improves motor fluctuations in levodopa-treated Parkinson's disease patients. Parkinson Study Group. Ann Neurol 1997;42:747–755.

39 Grill JD, Monsell SE: Choosing Alzheimer's disease prevention clinical trial populations. Neurobiol Aging 2014;35:466–471.

40 Chio A, Logroscino G, Hardiman O, et al: Prognostic factors in ALS: A critical review. Amyotroph Lateral Scler 2009; 10:310–323.

41 De Jager CA, Oulhaj A, Jacoby R, et al: Cognitive and clinical outcomes of homocysteine-lowering B-vitamin treatment in mild cognitive impairment: a randomized controlled trial. Int J Geriatr Psychiatry 2012;27:592–600.

42 Hartman JM, Forsen JW Jr, Wallace MS, et al: Tutorials in clinical research: part IV: recognizing and controlling bias. Laryngoscope 2002;112:23–31.

43 Baron S, Ulstein I, Werheid K: Psychosocial interventions in Alzheimer's disease and amnestic mild cognitive impairment: evidence for gender bias in clinical trials. Aging Ment Health 2015; 19:290–305.

44 Gwinn-Hardy K: Racial and ethnic influences on the expression of the genotype in neurodegenerative diseases; in Christen Y (ed): Genotype – Proteotype – Phenotype Relationships in Neurodegenerative Diseases. Paris, Springer, 2005, pp 27–36.

45 Risch N, Burchard E, Ziv E, et al: Categorization of humans in biomedical research: genes, race and disease. Genome Biol 2002;3:comment 2007.

46 Cosnett JE, Bill PL: Parkinson's disease in blacks. Observations on epidemiology in Natal. S Afr Med J 1988;73:281–283.

47 Chio A, Calvo A, Moglia C, et al: Phenotypic heterogeneity of amyotrophic lateral sclerosis: a population based study. J Neurol Neurosurg Psychiatry 2011;82: 740–746.

48 Guerchet M, Mouanga AM, M'belesso P, et al: Factors associated with dementia among elderly people living in two cities in Central Africa: the EDAC multicenter study. J Alzheimers Dis 2012;29:15–24.

49 Guerchet M, M'belesso P, Mouanga AM, et al: Prevalence of dementia in elderly living in two cities of Central Africa: the EDAC survey. Dement Geriatr Cogn Disord 2010;30:261–268.

50 Marin B, Logroscino G, Boumediene F, Labrunie A, Couratier P, Babron MC, Leutenegger AL, Preux PM, Beghi E: Clinical and demographic factors and outcome of amyotrophic lateral sclerosis in relation to population ancestral origin. Eur J Epidemiol 2016;31:229–245.

51 Marin B, Boumédiene F, Logroscino G, Couratier P, Babron MC, Leutenegger AL, Copetti M, Preux PM, Beghi E: Variation of amyotrophic lateral sclerosis's worldwide incidence – a meta-analysis. Int J Epidemiol 2016, in press.

52 Muangpaisan W, Hori H, Brayne C: Systematic review of the prevalence and incidence of Parkinson's disease in Asia. J Epidemiol 2009;19:281–293.

53 Lekoubou A, Echouffo-Tcheugui JB, Kengne AP: Epidemiology of neurodegenerative diseases in sub-Saharan Africa: a systematic review. BMC Public Health 2014;14:653.

54 Mukadam N, Cooper C, Livingston G: Improving access to dementia services for people from minority ethnic groups. Curr Opin Psychiatry 2013;26:409–414.

55 Chin AL, Negash S, Hamilton R: Diversity and disparity in dementia: the impact of ethnoracial differences in Alzheimer disease. Alzheimer Dis Assoc Disord 2011;25:187–195.

56 Sink KM, Covinsky KE, Newcomer R, et al: Ethnic differences in the prevalence and pattern of dementia-related behaviors. J Am Geriatr Soc 2004;52:1277–1283.

57 Marin B, Kacem I, Diagana M, et al: Juvenile and adult-onset ALS/MND among Africans: incidence, phenotype, survival: a review. Amyotroph Lateral Scler 2012;13:276–283.

58 Van Der Merwe C, Haylett W, Harvey J, et al: Factors influencing the development of early- or late-onset Parkinson's disease in a cohort of South African patients. S Afr Med J 2012;102:848–851.

59 Logroscino G, Traynor BJ, Hardiman O, et al: Incidence of amyotrophic lateral sclerosis in Europe. J Neurol Neurosurg Psychiatry 2010;81:385–390.

60 Del Aguila MA, Longstreth WT Jr, McGuire V, et al: Prognosis in amyotrophic lateral sclerosis: a population-based study. Neurology 2003;60:813–819.

61 Collomb H, Dumas M, Girard P: Neurological Disorders in Ghana. London, Oxford University Press, 1973.

62 Faison WE, Schultz SK, Aerssens J, et al: Potential ethnic modifiers in the assessment and treatment of Alzheimer's disease: challenges for the future. Int Psychogeriatr 2007;19:539–558.

63 Livney MG, Clark CM, Karlawish JH, et al: Ethnoracial differences in the clinical characteristics of Alzheimer's disease at initial presentation at an urban Alzheimer's disease center. Am J Geriatr Psychiatry 2011;19:430–439.

64 Renton AE, Chio A, Traynor BJ: State of play in amyotrophic lateral sclerosis genetics. Nat Neurosci 2014;17:17–23.

65 Yeo G: Ethnicity and dementia. J Am Geriatr Soc 2001;49:1393–1394.

66 Group UK-LS, Morrison KE, Dhariwal S, et al: Lithium in patients with amyotrophic lateral sclerosis (LiCALS): a phase 3 multicentre, randomised, double-blind, placebo-controlled trial. Lancet Neurol 2013;12:339–345.

67 Mizuno Y, Nomoto M, Kondo T, et al: Transdermal rotigotine in early stage Parkinson's disease: a randomized, double-blind, placebo-controlled trial. Mov Disord 2013;28:1447–1450.

68 Doody RS, Thomas RG, Farlow M, et al: Phase 3 trials of solanezumab for mild-to-moderate Alzheimer's disease. N Engl J Med 2014;370:311–321.

69 Sejvar JJ, Holman RC, Bresee JS, et al: Amyotrophic lateral sclerosis mortality in the United States, 1979–2001. Neuroepidemiology 2005;25:144–152.

70 Leone M, Chandra V, Schoenberg BS: Motor neuron disease in the United States, 1971 and 1973–1978: patterns of mortality and associated conditions at the time of death. Neurology 1987;37: 1339–1343.

71 Dean G, Quigley M, Goldacre M: Motor neuron disease in a defined English population: estimates of incidence and mortality. J Neurol Neurosurg Psychiatry 1994;57:450–454.

72 Mukadam N, Cooper C, Livingston G: A systematic review of ethnicity and pathways to care in dementia. Int J Geriatr Psychiatry 2011;26:12–20.

73 Venketasubramanian N, Sahadevan S, Kua EH, et al: Interethnic differences in dementia epidemiology: global and Asia-Pacific perspectives. Dement Geriatr Cogn Disord 2010;30:492–498.

74 Rochon PA, Berger PB, Gordon M: The evolution of clinical trials: inclusion and representation. CMAJ 1998;159:1373–1374.

75 Mckhann G, Drachman D, Folstein M, et al: Clinical diagnosis of Alzheimer's disease: report of the NINCDS-ADRDA Work Group under the auspices of Department of Health and Human Services Task Force on Alzheimer's Disease. Neurology 1984;34:939–944.

76 Hulley SB, Cummings SR, Browner WS, et al: Designing Clinical Research. Alphen aan den Rijn, Wolters Kluwer, Lippincot Williams and Wilkins, 2007.

77 Rollin-Sillaire A, Breuilh LJS, Salleron J, et al: Reason that prevent of Alzheimer's disease patients in clinical trials. Br J Clin Pharmacol 2013;75:1089–1097.

78 Bruandet A, Richard F, Bombois S, et al: Alzheimer disease with cerebrovascular disease and vascular dementia: clinical features and course compared with Alzheimer disease. J Neurol Neurosurg Psychiatry 2009;80:133–139.

79 Deschaintre Y, Richard F, Leys D, et al: Treatment of vascular risk factors is associated with slower decline in Alzheimer disease. Neurology 2009;73:674–680.

80 Rennie D: CONSORT revised – improving the reporting of randomized trials. JAMA 2001;285:2006–2007.

81 Juni P, Altman DG, Egger M: Systematic reviews in health care: assessing the quality of controlled clinical trials. BMJ 2001;323:42–46.

82 Begg C, Cho M, Eastwood S, et al: Improving the quality of reporting of randomized controlled trials. The CONSORT statement. JAMA 1996;276:637–639.

83 Moher D, Hopewell S, Schulz KF, et al: CONSORT 2010 explanation and elaboration: updated guidelines for reporting parallel group randomised trials. J Clin Epidemiol 2010;63:e1–e37.

84 Schriger DL, Arora S, Altman DG: The content of medical journal instructions for authors. Ann Emerg Med 2006;48:743–749.

85 Chan AW, Altman DG: Epidemiology and reporting of randomised trials published in PubMed journals. Lancet 2005;365:1159–1162.

86 86Hopewell S, Dutton S, Yu LM, et al: The quality of reports of randomised trials in 2000 and 2006: comparative study of articles indexed in PubMed. BMJ 2010;340:c723.

Giancarlo Logroscino
Unit of Neurodegenerative Diseases, Department of Clinical Research in Neurology
University of Bari 'Aldo Moro', 'Pia, Fondazione Cardinale G. Panico'
Via San Pio IX, n 4
IT–73039 Tricase (Italy)
E-Mail giancarlo.logroscino@uniba.it

Beghi E, Logroscino G (eds): The Right Therapy for Neurological Disorders. From Randomized Trials to Clinical Practice.
Front Neurol Neurosci. Basel, Karger, 2016, vol 39, pp 37–49 (DOI: 10.1159/000445411)

How to Distinguish between Statistically Significant Results and Clinically Relevant Results

Derrick A. Bennett

Clinical Trial Service Unit and Epidemiological Studies Unit, Nuffield Department of Population Health, University of Oxford, Oxford, UK

Abstract

Background: A practicing clinician will often be confronted with the results of a new clinical trial in their relevant field and will be faced with the dilemma of determining whether these results are clinically relevant to their own work. This chapter aims to describe the concepts of statistical significance in randomized clinical trials from a mainly classical statistical inference perspective. This chapter describes approaches to assess clinical significance and illustrates these approaches with examples from the contemporary neurological literature. ***Results:*** There are several approaches that have been described in the research literature to assess the clinical significance including the minimal important clinical difference, the fragility index, Bayesian approaches, and a graphical approach. Unfortunately none of these methods have been widely used in the neurological research literature. Examples are provided to illustrate how these methods can be applied to the contemporary neurological literature in order to provide the clinician with some guidance on their use. ***Conclusions:*** How the trial is designed can affect the external validity of the results and subsequently the clinical relevance of a randomized clinical trial. Large-scale streamlined clinical trials with inclusion criteria that are not too restrictive can improve the generalizability of trial results. Even highly statistically significant treatment effects can be unreliable if they are based on a small number of events. The approaches described in this chapter should provide the practicing clinician with a starting point in order to determine whether the reported statistically significant results are indeed clinically relevant.

Statistical thinking is an integral part of the research process in many scientific disciplines. A good understanding of statistics is relevant for defining the research question, design of the study, data collection, processing, and analysis through to interpretation and presentation of the results. In order to be as effective as possible, health professionals need to be able to read and evaluate the findings produced by research in their chosen field. Thus, a good grasp of the key statistical concepts is crucial for critically appraising the evidence and being able to put that evidence into practice. This chapter is split into four sections. First, a brief overview of statistical inference and its role in medical research are described. Second, an outline of the role of the randomized clinical trial (RCT) in medical research and why such study designs are the best way to assess causality is discussed. Third, the issue of generalizability (external validity) of an RCT is discussed and potential design issues that could make it difficult to apply the results of an RCT to clinical practice are described. Fourth, some approaches from the literature that aim to assess the clinical significance of RCT results are discussed with examples of trials from the neurological literature. The ultimate goal is to provide the readers with the basic tools to improve their ability to assess the clinical relevance of published neurological trials in relation to their patients and to public health in general.

Classical Statistical Inference

Classical statistical inference involves drawing conclusions about a population on the basis of a sample of the population. The two most common forms are hypothesis testing and estimation (confidence intervals).

Hypothesis Testing
A hypothesis is some testable belief or opinion, and hypothesis testing is the formal process by which statistical methods are used to assess the plausibility of this belief or opinion. Hypothesis testing attempts to measure the strength of evidence based on the sample of data concerning the research question of interest. The *null hypothesis* (denoted H_0) is often the negation of the research question that generated the data. In medical research where comparisons are being made between treatments or different groups of patients, the null hypothesis is that the 'true effect' of interest in the population is often zero or unity. The *alternative hypothesis* is usually the opposite of

the null hypothesis, e.g. that the 'true effect' of interest in the population is not zero. The alternative hypothesis (denoted H_1 or H_a) can on occasion specify that the 'true effect' in the population falls in one direction, e.g. that the true effect is greater than zero or unity or that that the true effect is less than zero or unity.

A *one-sided* alternative hypothesis is used when the direction of effect is specified. A *two-sided* test is used when no direction of effect is specified (i.e. the 'true effect' could be greater or less than the hypothesized value) [1]. There are only four possible results when we test a given hypothesis.
(1) We accept a true hypothesis – a correct decision
(2) We reject a true null hypothesis – an incorrect decision (type I error)
(3) We reject a false hypothesis – a correct decision
(4) We accept a false null hypothesis – an incorrect decision (type II error)

It is not possible to make a correct decision with 100% certainty when a hypothesis is tested via sampling and there is always the possibility of type I or II errors. In the statistical literature the probability of a type I error is denoted by α and the probability of a type II error is denoted β.

Significance Levels
Statistical significance measures how likely it is that any apparent differences in the observed sample data (e.g. in outcome between treatment and control groups) are real and not due to chance. The comparison of the test statistic from a statistical test with the appropriate distribution will return a p value, which will indicate the probability of obtaining a value as large as or more extreme than the test statistic when the null hypothesis is true.

The p value is usually compared to some selected cut-off value known as a significance level. The cut-off value for statistical significance in most medical studies is conventionally taken as 0.05 (5% significance level). The hypothesis test

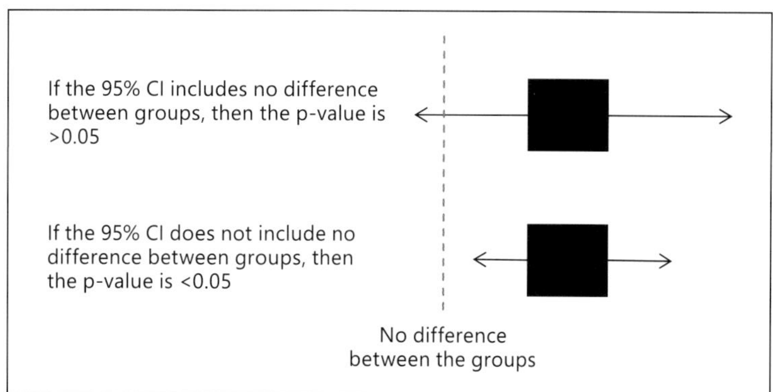

Fig. 1. Relationship between p value and 95% CI. Redrawn and adapted from [43].

aims to assess whether the difference between the hypothesis and the sample data can be attributed to random (chance) factors or not. If the hypothesis test indicates that the effect is probably not due to chance factors, then the null hypothesis can be rejected and the result is said to be statistically significant (p < 0.05). Although the 5% significance level is conventionally used in the medical literature depending on the nature of the study question, the p value may need to be much smaller than 0.05 before the study results can be considered to provide strong evidence against the null hypothesis in many situations [2].

Confidence Intervals
Confidence intervals estimate the range within which the real results would fall if the study was conducted many times. Specifically, the 95% confidence interval (CI) of the difference in treatment outcomes between two groups would indicate the range which the differences between the two treatments would fall on 95% of the occasions, if the study was carried out many times [3]. So, if the study was conducted on 20 occasions, then in 1 out of the 20 occasions the 95% CI would not contain the 'true effect' size just by chance. Hypothesis testing and confidence interval approaches to classical statistical inference are complementary as shown in figure 1. If the hypothesis test concludes that there is no difference between the two groups, the 95% CI would contain the 'no

difference' value and the p value would be greater than 0.05. Conversely, if the hypothesis test concludes that there 'is a difference' between the two groups, the 95% CI would exclude the 'no difference' value and the p value would be less than 0.05.

Bayesian Statistical Inference

The Bayesian paradigm differs from the classical statistical inference paradigm in that the uncertainty about an unknown parameter (e.g. a treatment effect) is expressed through an entire distribution called the prior distribution [4]. The prior distribution for the treatment effect expresses the prior uncertainty about the size of the treatment effect before collecting the data for the study. The basis of Bayesian statistical inference is to revise the estimate of the treatment effect based on the prior information to obtain a posterior distribution of the treatment effect [4, 5].

A major consideration of Bayesian statistical inference is the choice of the prior distribution. If there is not much prior information available, then a non-informative (sometimes called a vague, flat, or reference prior) can be used and this will have a minimal impact on the overall Bayesian analysis [6]. Information regarding the likely treatment effect and the uncertainty in this prior information may be obtained from the medical literature, pilot studies, or elicited from recognized experts in the relevant clinical area of interest. However, it is crucial that a wide range of experts are consulted to elicit prior information in order to encapsulate or represent a range of points of view, so that the uncertainty in their estimates is fully appreciated [7]. The posterior estimate contains the information from both the prior estimate and the findings of the new study. The posterior estimate enables the assessment of a range for the treatment effect, but there is no arbitrary cut-off whereby the study results are deemed positive or negative. This contrasts with classical hypothesis testing, in which a p value of 0.049 may be considered positive (i.e. statistically significant at the conventional 5% level), whereas a p value of 0.051 may be considered negative (i.e. statistically non-significant at the conventional 5% level) [7]. Several authors have proposed that more widespread use of Bayesian statistics would prevent the mistaken interpretation of p < 0.05 as showing that the null hypothesis is unlikely to be true and suggest that the adoption of these approaches would greatly improve the quality of medical research [8, 9]. We have already mentioned in the previous section that confidence intervals may be calculated in a classical analysis, but confidence intervals derived from a Bayesian analyses have a slightly different interpretation to the classical confidence interval and are called credible intervals. A 95% CI is one that has a 95% chance of containing the true population parameter of interest (e.g. treatment effect) [2, 4].

Introduction to Randomized Clinical Trials

RCTs are considered to be the most robust study design for assessing causality in medical research [10]. For example, in the simplest parallel group design to test the efficacy of a novel drug in the treatment of a specific disease, some patients with the disease are given the new drug and some are given the best existing drug. The two groups are then compared prospectively for incidence of disease and other important outcomes (also known as endpoints) of interest. Briefly, a high-quality RCT needs to utilize the following principles [11]:

(1) Proper randomization (allocation to the particular drug is done by a probabilistic random process that ensures balance for known and unknown factors)
(2) Minimize bias (patients, clinicians, and outcome evaluators should be unaware of the treatment allocation to the particular drug, and an adequate comparator group should be used)
(3) Intention-to-treat analyses (the treatment efficacy is based treatment allocated rather than treatment received, i.e. is the statistical analyses are performed according to the randomized groups regardless of adherence)
(4) Minimize the number of data-driven subgroup analyses (analysing many subgroups can produce chance results)

RCT Useful Metrics
Relative risks (RR) are independent of the prevalence of the disease and can be applied to populations with different prevalence of the disease. The RR is the ratio of the risks in the treatment group to the event rate in the control group. The absolute risk reduction (ARR) is the difference between the treatment group event rate and the control group event rate. The ARR and the derived metric 1/AAR known as the number needed to treat (NNT) vary with the prevalence of the disease. NNT is the number of patients needed to treat to prevent one adverse event, and the converse is known as the number needed to harm [12].

When reading the results of a study, the reader will need to consider the point estimate and confidence interval reported. Figure 2 shows the hypothetical results of three intervention studies. Study A suggests that the intervention has no effect (i.e. the true RR is 1) and is very precise (i.e.

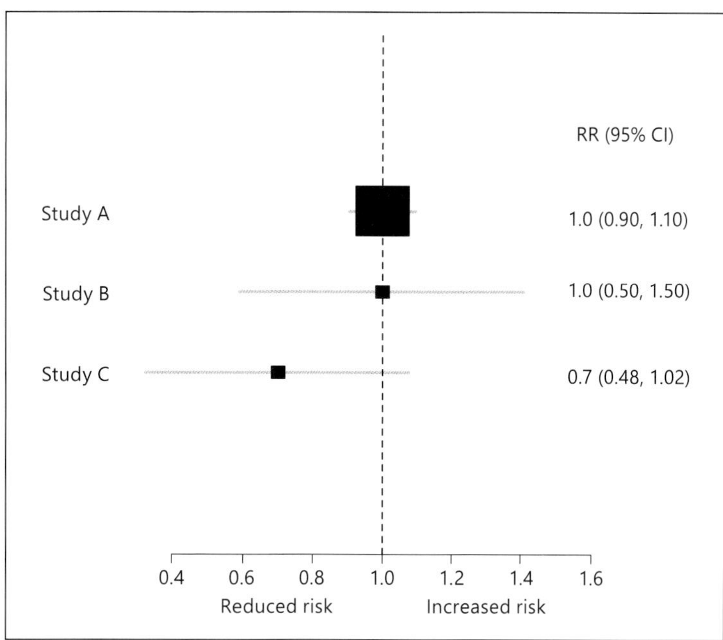

Fig. 2. Role of 95% CI in assessing type II errors. Redrawn and adapted from [44].

the confidence interval is narrow). You can be confident that it is not missing an important difference. Study B suggests that the intervention has no effect (i.e. the true RR is 1) but is very imprecise (i.e. the confidence interval is wide). This study may be missing an important difference. An investigator should be worried about a type II error, but this study is just as likely to be missing an important harmful effect as an important beneficial one. Study C suggests that the intervention has a potentially clinically important beneficial effect (i.e. the true RR is much less than 1) and is also very imprecise. A large part of the confidence interval includes potentially clinically important beneficial effects. As a consequence of this, an investigator might be concerned that a type II error is very likely. This is a study that should be repeated using a larger sample.

Care should be taken when interpreting non-statistically significant results such as those of study B in figure 2. It is quite common for investigators to confuse 'absence of evidence of effectiveness' with 'evidence of absence of effectiveness' [13]. For example, suppose a small trial is conducted to investigate the effect of a drug on death or dependency after stroke. Nine of 20 patients treated with drug are dead or dependent at follow-up compared with 10 of 20 untreated patients, giving a p value of 0.8. The absolute treatment effect is 5% (10/20 minus 9/20) with a 95% CI of 24, 33%. Based on this, it is plausible that the drug could cause either substantial harm or substantial benefit, so regardless of the p value the conclusion should be that there is still uncertainty about whether the drug works and a much larger trial is required in order to answer this research question reliably [14].

RCT Size

Given the side effects, costs, and inconveniences of a treatment, the minimal clinically important difference (MCID) is the smallest treatment efficacy that would lead to a change in a patient's management. The MCID is crucial in both planning of clinical trials and interpretation of their results. Sample size of a study is extremely important because if a study is too small, then it is unlikely that the investigators will be able to detect a modest, but clinically important, difference [10]. Conversely, if a study is too large, then time and resources will be wasted. Prior to the commencement of a study, the investigators should therefore spend time carefully deciding on a feasible sample size required in order to meet the goals of the study. The required sample size for a study depends on four criteria:

(1) The MCID that you wish to detect for the endpoint of interest
(2) The required power of the study (usually set at 80 or 90%)
(3) The required significance level (usually set at 5%)
(4) The variance of the endpoint or outcome of interest

The power of a test is 1 – probability of a type II error (i.e. $1 - \beta$). There are many different formulae for computing the required sample size which depend on the design of the study and the nature of the endpoint under study (e.g. time to event or dead or alive) [15]. For both standard errors and confidence intervals it is possible to increase precision by collecting a larger sample. Larger studies provide more precise estimates of effect size than small trials, and they may allow a few sensible and predefined subgroup analyses. Small studies, with wide confidence intervals around the effect size estimate are likely to be clinically uninformative (although they may add to a meta-analysis of all similar studies or generate enthusiasm for further investigation in a larger study) [14]. In a systematic review of the literature, Hislop et al. [16] found that there were a variety of methods available for specifying the MCID target difference in an RCT sample size calculation. The choice of approach was dependent on the aim (e.g. specifying an important difference versus a realistic difference), context (e.g. research question and availability of relevant data), and underlying framework adopted for the statistical analysis (e.g. classical statistical approach vs. Bayesian methods). They concluded that no single method provided an ideal solution for all contexts [16].

Generalizability or External Validity of a Randomized Clinical Trial

The practicing clinician would like to know if the results of an RCT are applicable to their patients. The results are likely to be 'clinically relevant' if the patients included in the trial were similar to those who would be treated in practice. Thus, if a treatment has only been tested in men aged under 40 years, then it is generally impossible to know if it will be of benefit to a woman aged over 65 years [17]. Usually, trials with broad inclusion criteria are more generalizable than those with very strict criteria. It should be possible by examining the inclusion and exclusion criteria and the baseline characteristics in the published trial report whether the trial sample is representative of the people a clinician wishes to treat in their own work [18]. However, it is important that the main emphasis of a trial's results should be placed on the overall effect and not on particular subgroups in the trial, especially if these subgroups have not been pre-specified beforehand [10, 14, 19].

Threats to the Generalizability of an RCT
There is often concern about the generalizability of trials done in secondary or tertiary care to practice in primary care. Differences in the health care system can affect external validity. Even if the health care systems are similar, other national differences can still affect generalizability [20]. For example, with cerebrovascular disease there are many important differences between countries in methods of diagnosis and management, as well as important racial differences in susceptibility to disease and natural history of the disease – all of which could affect the external validity of the trial results [17, 20]. Selection of participating centres from secondary care as opposed to primary care

has obvious implications for external validity, but RCTs of interventions that are confined to secondary care may also be undermined if they are restricted to specialist units. RCTs that have been conducted in a particular country will usually be generalizable to others, but this generalizability should not be taken for granted [17, 20].

Outcome Measures and Follow-Up

The external validity of an RCT also depends on whether the outcomes are clinically relevant. This can depend on who actually did the measurements, but is mostly dependent on what was measured and when [20]. RCTs sometimes use questionnaires, scales, or indexes that are often a mixture of symptoms and clinical signs. It is thus important to use validated and reliable questionnaires, scales, or indexes (with good repeatability and reproducibility) with clear definitions of what can be learned from absolute changes in the scale [21]. Many RCTs use composite outcome measures that can sometimes combine events of different severity and treatment effects can be driven by the least important outcome, which are often the most frequent events [20]. This is usually the situation in trials of stroke that include transient ischaemic attacks in a composite outcome. Inadequate duration of treatment and/or follow-up can also have an effect on the external validity of a trial [11]. For example, patients with Alzheimer's disease (AD) may require treatment for many years; however, most RCTs of new drugs in this area follow up the effects of treatment only for a few months or years [22].

Stopping a Clinical Trial Early

Some trials are planned to be much larger than the size of the study that is reported in the final published manuscript. Trials may end up smaller because they are stopped early due to an apparently substantial treatment benefit (stopping for efficacy). The results of such studies may need to be treated with a degree of scepticism because if they had been allowed to continue, the final esti-mated treatment effect may well have been much smaller, so the reported estimate may be an over-estimate of the treatment effect [23, 24]. In the very early stages of a trial, the treatment effect tends to fluctuate between extreme values before becoming more settled as more data accrues. Thus, trials that stop early may have just stopped on a random high or low [14]. Obviously, there can be strong ethical reasons why a trial may stop early, such as unexpected harmful effects [or no apparent emerging benefits (stopping for futility)]. However, the trial data monitoring committee needs to think carefully about the possibility that early harm may be outweighed by longer-term benefits later as more information becomes available [14, 25–27].

Approaches to Assess Clinical Significance

In classical statistical inference, statistical significance measures how likely is it that the observed differences in outcome between treatment and control groups are real and not due to the play of chance. Clinical significance measures how large the differences in effect size (e.g. RR, mean difference, or some other metric of interest) are in clinical practice. There have been several attempts in the literature to try and combine statistical and clinical significance in such a way the trial results can be interpreted more easily. These approaches are now described in more detail.

Using Minimal Clinically Important Difference in Order to Assess Clinical Significance

Man-Son-Hing et al. [28] have suggested that clinical importance can take four forms, depending on the relationship of the MCID of the intervention to the point estimate (the best single value of the efficacy of the intervention that has been derived from the study results) and the 95% CI surrounding it:

(1) Definite: when the MCID is smaller than the lower limit of the 95% CI

(2) Probable: when the MCID is greater than the lower limit of the 95% CI, but smaller than the point estimate of the efficacy of the intervention

(3) Possible: when the MCID is less than the upper limit of the 95% CI, but greater than the point estimate of the efficacy of the intervention

(4) Definitely not: when the MCID is greater than the upper limit of the 95% CI

These concepts are now illustrated using some examples from the contemporary neurological literature.

Study Results of Definite Clinical Importance

A study will have results of *definite clinical importance* if the lower limit of the 95% CI is greater than the MCID. Given that the 95% CI is greater than the MCID estimate, studies with definite clinical importance will always be statistically significant (p < 0.05). An example is the FREEDOMS II trial [29] that investigated the efficacy and safety of fingolimod (an oral sphingosine-1-phosphate receptor modulator that has shown reductions in clinical and MRI disease activity in patients with multiple sclerosis). The primary objective was to assess whether fingolimod 0.5 mg per day was superior to placebo in reducing annualized relapse rates in patients with relapsing-remitting multiple sclerosis treated for up to 24 months. The authors report that the MCID was to detect a relative annualized relapse rate reduction of 40% (i.e. they could detect a rate ratio of 0.60). Three hundred and fifty-eight patients were randomized to fingolimod and 355 to receive placebo. The mean annualized relapse rate was 0.40 (95% CI: 0.34, 0.48) in patients given placebo and 0.21 (95% CI: 0.17, 0.25) in patients given fingolimod 0.5 mg. This corresponded to a rate ratio of 0.52 (95% CI: 0.40, 0.66) and a p value of <0.0001 for fingolimod versus placebo.

Another example of such a result that was statistically significant is from the MEMREHAB trial, a double-blind placebo-controlled trial of 86 patients with definite multiple sclerosis [30]. The objective was to examine the efficacy of the modified Story Memory Technique (mSMT), a 10-session behavioural intervention teaching context and imagery to facilitate learning, to improve learning and memory in person with multiple sclerosis. Participants completed neuropsychological assessment at baseline, a repeat assessment immediately after treatment, and a long-term follow-up assessment at 6 months. After completion of the treatment phase, the participants were assigned to receive or not receive booster sessions, in order to assess the efficacy of monthly booster sessions. The authors reported a MCID of 0.13 in the learning slope for the California Verbal Learning test between the treatment and control group. The treatment group showed a significantly improved learning slope difference when compared to the placebo group after treatment of 0.54 (95% CI: 0.21, 0.87) with an associated p value of 0.021.

Study Results of Probable Clinical Importance

The results of a study that is of *probable clinical importance* will have 95% CIs that include the value of the MCID, with the point estimate being greater than the MCID estimate. The study results may or may not be statistically significant. An example from the neurological literature is the trials of amyotrophic lateral sclerosis (ALS), a progressive degenerative disease that is characterized by weakness in the limbs and bulbar muscles. The first trial in this area by Bensimon et al. [31] used a drug called riluzole in order to assess improved survival at 12 months in ALS compared with placebo. The authors reported a MCID of 30% improved survival at 12 months for patients with bulbar-onset disease for the basis of their sample size calculations. They found that 12-month survival was 35% in the placebo group versus 73% in the riluzole group (absolute reduction increase in survival of 38%), which was statistically significant with a p value of 0.014. The same trial also investigated patients with limb-onset ALS and found no significant improvement in survival at 12 months (p = 0.17). There was concern about the disproportionate benefit in the patients with bulbar-disease onset compared to lumbar disease-onset ALS. As this trial was relatively small (~150 patients), a much larger trial that varied the dosage of riluzole was carried out and this also found a small but statistically significant prolongation of survival in participants receiving the intermediate and high dose of riluzole [32]. Some patients were ineligible for the large trial and as a consequence another trial of riluzole was conducted (in parallel with the larger study) with patients with either more advanced ALS or aged over 75 years as the patient population. This study was not statistically significant, but the study was not designed to assess efficacy, so it did not demonstrate a survival advantage of riluzole. However, although not statistically significant, the result was of probable clinical importance as it did demonstrate that riluzole was well tolerated in this patient population, and that the adverse events were similar to those observed in the larger definitive trials [33].

Study Results of Possible Clinical Importance
Studies with results of possible clinical importance have 95% CIs that include the value of the MCID and an MCID greater than the efficacy point estimate. The results may or may not be statistically significant. An example of a study result that is of possible clinical importance that was not statistically significant is the URICO-ICTUS study [34]. This study aimed to assess whether uric acid therapy would improve functional outcomes at 90 days in patients with acute ischaemic stroke. The primary outcome was patients with an excellent outcome [i.e. a modified Rankin score (mRS) of 0–1, or 2 if the premorbid score was 2] at 90 days. The MCID was estimated to be a 14% difference between uric acid and placebo. Two hundred and eleven patients received uric acid and 200 received placebo; of these, 83 (39%) that received uric acid and 66 (33%) that received

placebo had an excellent outcome. The absolute treatment difference observed was 6% with an adjusted risk ratio of 0.81 (95% CI: 0.64, 1.04; p = 0.099).

Another example of a study result that is of possible clinical importance that was statistically significant is the TEAM-AD VA Cooperative randomized trial [35]. This study aimed to investigate whether vitamin E (α-tocopherol), memantine, or both slow progression of mild-to-moderate AD in patients taking an acetylcholinesterase inhibitor. The trial involved 613 patients with mild-to-moderate AD and 152 participants received α-tocopherol, 155 received memantine, 154 the combination of memantine and α-tocopherol, and 152 placebo. The MCID was a 4-point mean treatment difference in the Alzheimer's Disease Cooperative study Activities of Daily Living (ADCS-ADL) between either treatment given alone versus placebo. The MCID was also estimated as a 20% reduction in the annual rate of AD decline. Participants receiving α-tocopherol had a mean change difference compared with placebo of 3.15 (95% CI: 0.92, 5.39); the p value after adjustment was 0.03. This change translates into a delay in AD progression of 19% per year compared with placebo.

Study Results That Are Definitely Not Clinically Important
Studies that produce results that are definitely not of clinical importance have an upper limit of the 95% CI that is below the MCID. Again the study results may or may not be statistically significant. An example of a study result that was definitely not clinically important in the neurological literature that was also not statistically significant is the ALIAS trial [36], which aimed to assess whether albumin given within 5 h of the onset of acute ischaemic stroke increased the proportion of patients with a favourable outcome. The MCID reported by the authors was a 20% absolute difference between thrombolysis and non-thrombolysis strata. Four hundred and twenty-two patients

were randomized to receive albumin and 419 to receive saline. The trial was stopped early for futility with 814 patients recruited into the study. The primary outcome did not differ between the patients in the albumin and saline groups [186 (44%) vs. 185 (44%); risk ratio 0.96 (95% CI: 0.84, 1.10)].

An example of a statistically significant result that was definitely not of clinical importance was the GISSI-Prevenzione trial, which assessed the effects of dietary supplementation with polyunsaturated fats on death, non-fatal myocardial infarction, and non-fatal stroke [37]. The MCID was considered to be a 4% absolute reduction in deaths for the composite endpoints between the groups over a 3.5-year period. The study actually observed a 1.3% (95% CI: 0.1, 2.6) absolute reduction in the primary endpoint.

A Potential New Metric to Assess Clinical Significance
As has already been described, p values and 95% CI can be used to help determine how likely observed effects are on the basis of chance. Walsh et al. [38] proposed that in the case of RCTs with dichotomous outcomes, a shift of only a few events in one group could change typical hypothesis tests above the usual thresholds considered statistically significant (i.e. p < 0.05). They suggest a new approach that they feel can better communicate the limitations of p value thresholds as this new metric demonstrates how easily significance based on a threshold p value may be exceeded. They refer to this metric as a fragility index (FI). The FI helps to identify the number of events required to change statistically significant results to non-significant results.

We will illustrate the use of this metric using the GISSI-Prevenzione trial results. The study aimed to compare the effects of polyunsaturated fats (n-3-PUFA) versus placebo on the composite endpoint of death, non-fatal myocardial infarction, and non-fatal stroke in 11,324 patients [37]. The number of events in the n-3-PUFA group

Table 1. An example of fragility using data from the GISSI-Prevenzione trial

a Results

	Event	No event
n-3-PUFA	715	4,951
Control	785	4,883

RR = 0.90 (95% CI: 0.82, 1.00); Fisher's exact test = 0.05.

b Calculated fragility of the results

	Event	No event
n-3-PUFA	718	4,948
Control	785	4,883

RR = 0.90 (95% CI: 0.81, 1.01); Fisher's exact test = 0.06.

was 715 (21.6%) versus 785 (13.9%) in the placebo group with an RR of 0.90 (95% CI: 0.82, 0.99) and a corresponding value of 0.05. The results of the trial are presented as a two-by-two table with the number of events over the entire follow-up being used to construct the table (table 1a).

The FI is calculated by adding an event from the group with the smaller number of events (and subtracting the non-event from the same group to keep the total number of patients constant) and recalculating the two-sided p value for Fisher's exact test [38]. Table 1b shows the RR after adding 3 events to the n-3-PUFA event group (and subtracting 3 events from the non-event group to keep patient numbers constant). The RR is still 0.90, but Fisher's exact p value is 0.06. So it only took 3 events to change this result from significant to non-statistically significant at the conventional 5% level of significance. The importance of the FI can be appreciated if consideration is given to RCTs where initial reports showed statistically significant effects that were later shown to be either substantially less than previously reported or ineffective [39].

A Bayesian Approach to Clinical Significance
Burton et al. [40] describe a Bayesian approach to clinical significance. They report that their approach is most useful in situations in which a conventional classical statistical approach to the analysis may be difficult or misleading. They suggest that their approach includes circumstances in which: (1) a statistically non-significant result is large enough to be clinically relevant (small sample size), (2) a statistically significant result is too small to be of clinical relevance (very large sample size), or (3) it is desired that conclusions are drawn about the probable similarity of two outcomes without concluding that non-significant means that there is no difference. Although this Bayesian approach was first described almost two decades ago [40], it has not received widespread use in the neurological literature (probably due to the difficulty in eliciting prior information), where classical statistical approaches to statistical inference dominate in published reports.

A Graphical Approach to Clinical Significance
The level of treatment effect regarded as clinically significant also depends on the severity of the disease and any potential side effects of the treatment. As described earlier in this chapter, a common strategy to assess combined statistical and clinical significance is to report an appropriate metric (e.g. RR, ARR, or NNT) with its associated 95% CI. The levels of treatment effects regarded as clinically worthwhile are likely to differ among clinicians and settings. If one clinician considers that introduction of the new treatment is worthwhile only if the actual risk is reduced by 15%, it is important to know how likely the clinical trial observations would have arisen by chance with the null hypothesis that the new treatment has an ARR of less than 0.15 and not with the null hypothesis that the two treatments are equally effective. This leads to the Bayesian approach by Burton et al. [40] reported in the previous section. As an alternative, Leung [41] proposed a plot of p value-ARR or p value-NNT which he believes would be useful to the clinicians who practise evidence-based medicine. In the null hypothesis, the Leung approach assumes that the ARR for the new treatment is less than some value x. p values are calculated for a range of values of x. These p values are plotted on the vertical axis and the ARR on the horizontal axis. Hence, for a range of values of ARR, the plot will show the corresponding probability that the clinical trial observations would have arisen by chance if the real ARR were less than the given values [41]. This approach was described over a decade ago and as with the Bayesian approach [40], it has not been used at all in the neurological literature where classical statistical approaches still prevail in the interpretation of trial results.

Conclusion

This chapter aimed to give a general overview of the differences between statistical and clinical significance in the context of RCTs of neurological disorders. A description of the practical design issues that can affect the external validity and subsequently the clinical relevance of an RCT (e.g. the choice of the study population, outcome measures used, length of follow-up, sample size, and stopping a trial early) have also been provided. In addition, approaches that use the minimally important clinical difference with examples from the contemporary neurological literature have also been discussed in order to facilitate interpretation. Modest treatment effects on mortality or major morbidity are generally more plausible than large effects. It has often been the case that large and often striking effects from small-scale randomized trials (and other types of designs including non-randomized studies) will often be refuted [10, 42]. This implies that even highly statistically significant (e.g. 2-sided p values of 0.001) differences that are based on only relatively small numbers of events in selected studies may provide untrustworthy evidence of the existence of any real clinically important difference. Finally, when there is a lack of good evidence for any effect on major outcomes, estimates of the NNT to prevent such outcomes are of little or no value, and it is particularly important to provide confidence intervals around the NNT [12] in order that the range uncertainty can be ascertained. For this reason, based on classical statistical inference, statistically significant results with claims of large effects based on small randomized trials should be treated with caution by practicing clinicians until the clinical relevance can be reliably assessed.

References

1 Bland JM, Bland DG: One and two sided tests of significance. BMJ 1994;309:248.

2 Sterne JAC, Cox DR, Smith GD: Sifting the evidence – what's wrong with significance tests? Another comment on the role of statistical methods. BMJ 2001;322:226–231.

3 Gardener M, Altman D: Confidence intervals rather than p values: estimation rather than hypothesis testing. Br Med J (Clin Res Ed) 1986;292:746–750.

4 Berry DA: Introduction to Bayesian methods III: use and interpretation of Bayesian tools in design and analysis. Clin Trials 2005;2:295–300.

5 Spiegelhalter DJ, Myles JP, Jones DR, Abrams KR: An introduction to Bayesian methods in health technology assessment. BMJ 1999;319:508–512.

6 Ibrahim JG, Chen M-H, Chu H: Bayesian methods in clinical trials: a Bayesian analysis of ECOG trials E1684 and E1690. BMC Med Res Methodol 2012; 12:183.

7 Lewis RJ, Wears RL: An introduction to the Bayesian analysis of clinical trials. Ann Emerg Med 1993;22:1328–1336.

8 Lilford RJ, Braunholtz D: For Debate: The statistical basis of public policy: a paradigm shift is overdue. BMJ 1996; 313:603–607.

9 Carlin BP, Louis TA: Bayesian Methods for Data Analysis. Boca Raton, Hall/ CRC, 2008.

10 Collins R, MacMahon S: Reliable assessment of the effects of treatment on mortality and major morbidity, I: clinical trials. Lancet 2001;357:373–380.

11 Baigent C, Peto R, Gray R, Parish S, Collins R: Large-Scale Randomized Evidence: Trials and Meta-Analyses of Trials. Oxford, Oxford University Press, 2010, pp 31–45.

12 Altman DG: Confidence intervals for the number needed to treat. BMJ 1998;317: 1309–1312.

13 Altman DG, Bland JM: Absence of evidence is not evidence of absence. BMJ 1995;311:485.

14 Lewis SC, Warlow CP: How to spot bias and other potential problems in randomised controlled trials. J Neurol Neurosurg Psychiatry 2004;75:181–187.

15 Wittes J: Sample size calculations for randomized controlled trials. Epidemiol Rev 2002;24:39–53.

16 Hislop J, Adewuyi TE, Vale LD, et al: Methods for specifying the target difference in a randomised controlled trial: the Difference ELicitation in TriAls (DELTA) systematic review. PLoS Med 2014;11:e1001645.

17 Altman DG, Bland JM: Generalisation and extrapolation. BMJ 1998;317:409– 410.

18 Schulz KF, Grimes DA: Sample size slippages in randomised trials: exclusions and the lost and wayward. Lancet 2002; 359:781–785.

19 Rothwell PM: Treating individuals 2. Subgroup analysis in randomised controlled trials: importance, indications, and interpretation. Lancet 2005;365: 176–186.

20 Rothwell PM: External validity of randomised controlled trials: 'to whom do the results of this trial apply?' Lancet 2005;365:82–93.

21 Bland JM, Altman DG: Validating scales and indexes. BMJ 2002;324:606–607.

22 Kryscio RJ: Secondary prevention trials in Alzheimer disease: the challenge of identifying a meaningful end point. JAMA Neurol 2014;71:947–949.

23 Guyatt GH, Briel M, Glasziou P, Bassler D, Montori VM: Problems of stopping trials early. BMJ 2012;344:e3863.

24 Bassler D, Briel M, Montori VM, et al: Stopping randomized trials early for benefit and estimation of treatment effects: systematic review and meta-regression analysis. JAMA 2010;303: 1180–1187.

25 Grant AM, Altman DG, Babiker AB, et al: Issues in data monitoring and interim analysis of trials. Health Technol Assess 2005;9:1–238, iii–iv.

26 Bassler D, Montori VM, Briel M, Glasziou P, Guyatt G: Early stopping of randomized clinical trials for overt efficacy is problematic. J Clin Epidemiol 2008; 61:241–246.

27 Chalmers I, Altman DG, McHaffie H, Owens N, Cooke RW: Data sharing among data monitoring committees and responsibilities to patients and science. Trials 2013;14:102.

28 Man-Son-Hing M, Laupacis A, O'Rourke K, et al: Determination of the clinical importance of study results. J Gen Intern Med 2002;17:469–476.

29 Calabresi PA, Radue E-W, Goodin D, et al: Safety and efficacy of fingolimod in patients with relapsing-remitting multiple sclerosis (FREEDOMS II): a double-blind, randomised, placebo-controlled, phase 3 trial. Lancet Neurol 2014;13:545–556.

30 Chiaravalloti ND, Moore NB, Nikelshpur OM, DeLuca J: An RCT to treat learning impairment in multiple sclerosis: the MEMREHAB trial. Neurology 2013;81:2066–2072.

31 Bensimon G, Lacomblez L, Meininger VA: Controlled trial of riluzole in amyotrophic lateral sclerosis. N Engl J Med 1994;330:585–591.

32 Lacomblez L, Bensimon G, Meininger V, Leigh PN, Guillet P: Dose-ranging study of riluzole in amyotrophic lateral sclerosis. Amyotrophic Lateral Sclerosis/Riluzole Study Group II. Lancet 1996;347: 1425–1431.

33 Bensimon G, Lacomblez L, Delumeau JC, Bejuit R, Truffinet P, Meininger V: A study of riluzole in the treatment of advanced stage or elderly patients with amyotrophic lateral sclerosis. J Neurol 2002;249:609–615.

34 Chamorro Á, Amaro S, Castellanos M, et al: Safety and efficacy of uric acid in patients with acute stroke (URICO-ICTUS): a randomised, double-blind phase 2b/3 trial. Lancet Neurol 2014;13: 453–460.

35 Dysken MW, Sano M, Asthana S, et al: Effect of vitamin E and memantine on functional decline in Alzheimer disease: The TEAM-AD VA cooperative randomized trial. JAMA 2014;311:33–44.

36 Ginsberg MD, Palesch YY, Hill MD, et al: High-dose albumin treatment for acute ischaemic stroke (ALIAS) part 2: a randomised, double-blind, phase 3, placebo-controlled trial. Lancet Neurol 2013;12:1049–1058.

37 Dietary supplementation with n-3 polyunsaturated fatty acids and vitamin E after myocardial infarction: results of the GISSI-Prevenzione trial. Lancet 1999;354:447–455.

38 Walsh M, Srinathan SK, McAuley DF, et al: The statistical significance of randomized controlled trial results is frequently fragile: a case for a fragility index. J Clin Epidemiol 2014;67:622–628.

39 Ioannidis JA: Contradicted and initially stronger effects in highly cited clinical research. JAMA 2005;294:218–228.

40 Burton PR, Gurrin LC, Campbell MJ: Clinical significance not statistical significance: a simple Bayesian alternative to p values. J Epidemiol Community Health 1998;52:318–323.

41 Leung WC: Balancing statistical and clinical significance in evaluating treatment effects. Postgrad Med J 2001;77: 201–204.

42 Ioannidis JPA: Why most published research findings are false. PLoS Med 2005;2:e124.

43 Primer on 95% confidence intervals. Eff Clin Pract 2001;4:229–231.

44 Primer on Type 1 and Type II errors. Eff Clin Pract 2001;4:284–285.

Derrick A. Bennett, PhD
Clinical Trial Service Unit and Epidemiological Studies Unit
Nuffield Department of Population Health, Old Road Campus
Roosevelt Drive, Headington
Oxford OX3 7LF (UK)
E-Mail derrick.bennett@ctsu.ox.ac.uk

Beghi E, Logroscino G (eds): The Right Therapy for Neurological Disorders. From Randomized Trials to Clinical Practice.
Front Neurol Neurosci. Basel, Karger, 2016, vol 39, pp 50–59 (DOI: 10.1159/000445412)

Modeling and Prediction in Neurological Disorders: The Biostatistical Perspective

Massimiliano Copetti[a] · Andrea Fontana[a] · Fabio Pellegrini[b]

[a] Unit of Biostatistics, IRCSS Casa Sollievo della Sofferenza, San Giovanni Rotondo, Italy; [b] Worldwide Medical, Biogen Idec Inc., Cambridge, Mass., USA

Abstract

Background: Statistical methods are often considered as mere tools to address research questions. The lack of critical understanding can make their use sometimes highly questionable if not inappropriate. Biostatistics should be seen more as a paradigm than a set of tools. Knowledge of methods means a flexible utilization of them, in which modeling and prediction correspond more to an art than to a routine use dictated by circumstances and habits. ***Summary:*** Tree-based methods (or tree-growing techniques) are discussed here as a flexible statistical framework for modeling and prediction to address key questions such as prognostic stratification and treatment effects heterogeneity in both randomized clinical trials and observational studies. ***Key Messages:*** We provide some examples in neurology and possible future extensions in which tree-based methods are shown to be crucial for the assessment of the best available therapy for a patient. We show how trees can represent a clinically interpretable and easy-to-implement approach for stratified medicine and treatment tailoring based on responsiveness, as well as for selecting populations for new studies.

A Rationale for Stratified Medicine

Statistical modeling and prediction play a fundamental role in the understanding of randomized clinical trials. Whether or not a randomized clinical trial will be a success is strictly connected to the soundness of its clinical and methodological bases. The starting point of our discussion is focused on a specific task biostatistics can serve: how statistical modeling and prediction can help in phase III trial failures.

The understanding of why phase III trials in some neurological disorders have failed to prove efficacy [1] needs a solid reassessment from a methodological perspective. Basically three major concerns summarize the problem of phase III failure: Was the phase II trial conducted on a sufficiently large sample size and the primary end point assessed over an adequately long follow-up time so as to justify a phase III trial? Was the primary end point sensitive to capture treatment response? And, was the target population appropriately selected?

The purpose of this chapter is to provide some answers to the latter two questions and a viable path for designing future trials minimizing the risk of failure. An answer to the first question needs a different focus and is beyond the scope of this chapter.

First of all, in our view, more consideration should be given to the understanding of the disease course. That is, what are the prognostic factors for the end point in the placebo arm? This – as we will see later – is essential to tailor the actual population we intend to use in a trial.

When a complex or heterogeneous pattern of prognosis underlies the disease, particular care should be taken from a methodological standpoint to address this concern. Stratified medicine is not merely a fashionable topic, but addresses most of the hidden issues of lack of efficacy in phase III trials. A fundamental review paper on this topic has been recently published in neurology [2], although – surprisingly – it does not directly address amyotrophic lateral sclerosis (ALS), which occupies a particular place for unsuccessful phase III trial attempts [1].

Given the disease, stratified medicine allows to assess the existence of population subgroups according to differences in prognosis and treatment response [3]. The difference can rely on clinical and demographical characteristics, genetic background, and biomarkers. A clear distinction is necessary to understand whether such aspects represent prognostic factors and/or treatment effect modifiers [3]. A patient's characteristics such as age, gender, disease duration, etc., is defined as a prognostic factor when its variability determines different outcomes of prognosis over time, whereas the same characteristic is called a treatment effect modifier (i.e. affects the response to treatment) when its variability significantly determines different outcomes of treatment efficacy [3].

It is fundamental to understand that if some effect modifiers are present within the target population of a trial which failed to yield an overall significant finding, the chances to miss a significant result in one or more subgroups are non-null. This is especially true when effect modifiers are qualitative and not quantitative, i.e. when treatment effects show opposite signs between the subgroups or strata determined by the modifier itself. However, first of all, we must go back to understand the potential prognostic stratification in the control arm.

Prognosis and Treatment-by-Covariate Interactions via Tree-Based Methods

Interesting approaches have been recently developed, even in the context of individual patient data mixed treatment comparisons, where most of the attention has shifted to subgroup comparisons driven by additive or multiplicative multivariable regression [4–6] and by tree-based methods [7, 8]. Here we will discuss the approach based on tree-growing techniques, introducing the rationale for prognostic stratification and treatment-by-covariate interaction detection, i.e. differential response to treatment.

This approach is not new and has recently received renewed attention [9]. Moreover, some authors for the first time have provided a generalization of tree-based methods to select a target population for future clinical trials [10, 11]. The understanding of prognostic stratification and treatment responsiveness are indeed the two main aspects of population targeting for clinical trials. A novel temptation which we fear could be somehow misleading in the process of selecting a promising population for a new phase III trial is to use the so-called 'interaction trees', i.e. trees which directly test and stratify the sample analyzed according to heterogeneous treatment effects, immaterial of the prognostic role of the same strata.

We advocate, as for an alternative sound approach not based on trees [6], that the first step should always consist of analyzing the prognosis

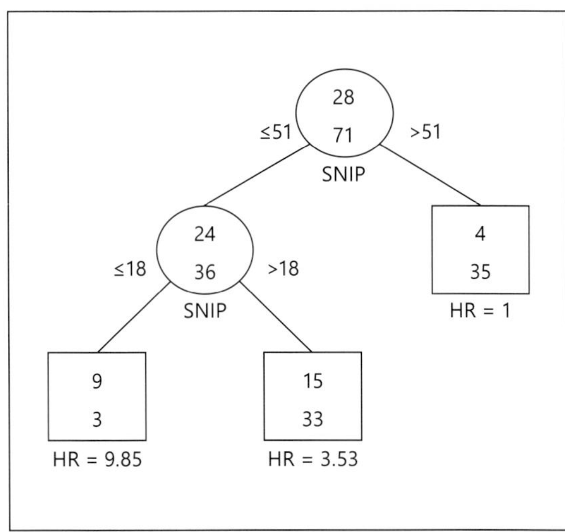

Fig. 1. A tree-structured representation for the risk of tracheostomy or death in a sample of ALS patients. The RECPAM tree-growing algorithm (see [12]) estimates risks from a Cox proportional hazards regression model, where sex, Amyotrophic Lateral Sclerosis Functional Rating Scale revisited, site of the onset, forced vital capacity, and SNIP were considered candidate splitting variables. Age at the first visit, Charlson Comorbidity Index, and disease duration (for each unitary increase of 5 years) were used as global adjustment variables. Selected splitting variables are shown between branches, while the condition sending patients to the left or right subgroup is on a relative branch. Results are reported as hazard ratios (HR). The subgroup with the lowest event rate was considered as the reference category (HR = 1). Numbers inside circles and squares represent the number of events (top) and the number of nonevents (bottom), respectively.

in the control arm since any specific benefit of treatment will be potentially conditioned by the event rate in each subgroup (i.e. a higher event rate in the control arm gives more chance for a larger treatment effect), and that response to treatment should be investigated along with prognosis and not separately. Indeed, a tree can express a prognostic gradient of the strata plus the specific role of treatment within each subgroup [12] formalized in one single equation in which the prognostic gradient simply corresponds to the contrasts of subgroup-specific intercepts.

The risk stratification process that a tree represents is known under different names: recursive partitioning algorithms, tree-growing techniques, tree-structured regression, and tree-based methods [9]. Many approaches are now widespread and commercial software or macro routines in R are available [8–11]. GUIDE (Generalized Unbiased Interaction Detection and Estimation) [8], SIDES (Subgroup Identification based on Differential Effect Search) [10], and RECPAM (Recursive Partitioning and Amalgamation) [12] will be our reference approaches here. For a general review of tree-growing techniques the reader is referred elsewhere [9].

A tree is a simple graphical display of the relationship between a set of user-defined candidate covariates or predictors and an outcome (fig. 1). The display must be read from top to bottom in its process of recursive stratification of the covariate space. Each subgroup is represented by a circle called a 'node', whereas squares represent final subgroups and are named 'leaves'. Nodes can be connected top-down to reach leaves; therefore, a connection line (i.e. a 'branch') defines a parent-child relationship, and nodes or leaves on the same level can be also called 'siblings'. Usually the variable determining the stratification for each node is placed under the node itself, and the left and right subgroup assignment rules (i.e. 'conditions') are reported on each branch.

Typically, as in our example in figure 1, nodes and leaves report inside the number of events (top) and nonevents (bottom); however, according to the type of outcome, the total number of subjects, mean values, proportions, rates, or any other subgroup-level summary statistics could be reported as well. Each leaf commonly displays a summary expression of the relative risk (namely hazard ratios in fig. 1), setting the rightmost leaf (that with the lowest incidence) as the reference category. When interaction trees are displayed, a leaf-specific measure of relative risk (treatment vs. placebo) is reported as well. Further clarifying details are provided in the legend of figure 1 below.

Prognostic stratification via a recursive partitioning method is carried out maximizing between-subgroups heterogeneity with respect to the outcome. A splitting function is used to capture the degree of heterogeneity and is commonly defined as a separation function or, simply, as deviance or a χ^2 test. The partitioning algorithm recursively searches through all the covariates considered for the analysis and all the potential cutoff points, and stops when a predefined number of interaction levels or a minimum sample size is reached. An a posteriori stratification, therefore, is derived from the original sample, where only variables that play a statistically and/or clinically significant role are stratified for.

A key feature of tree modeling is the 'pruning' step to avoid overfitting and to obtain a stable structured set of predictors. Tree pruning is commonly pursued in most of the approaches through cross-validation [8, 10, 12]. Some methods, such as RECPAM, also include an amalgamation step, in which nonsibling leaves may be collapsed again according to a deviance test for information content loss [12]. This feature is seldom used though clinically intriguing, and intuitively consists of merging different covariate interaction patterns (classes) that have almost overlapping risks. Therefore, not only is risk stratification possible (prognostic trees), but covariate-treatment interaction detection is also assessable (interaction or predictive trees) [10]. In this case, the partitioning algorithm recursively searches within the candidate covariates for the two subgroups in which the heterogeneity in treatment effect is maximized.

A simple prognostic tree with two leaves for a binary outcome with probability p is of the form:

$$\text{logit}(p) = \beta_0 + \beta_1 X \qquad (1)$$

while a predictive tree is:

$$\text{logit}(p) = \beta_0 + \beta_1 X + \beta_2 Z \cdot I_{[X=0]} + \beta_3 Z \cdot I_{[X=1]} \qquad (2)$$

In equations 1 and 2, where for the sake of simplicity X represents a binary baseline covariate, Z a binary treatment, and I the indicator function, β_0 corresponds to the logit transformation for the probability p of the outcome in the prognostic subgroup X = 0, whereas $\beta_0 + \beta_1$ identifies the logit transformation for the probability p in the prognostic subgroup X = 1. Straightforwardly, e^{β_1} is the odds ratio between the two prognostic classes. Furthermore, in 2, e^{β_2} and e^{β_3} are the odds ratios for treatment versus placebo within the two specific prognostic classes, respectively. In equation 2 the picture is now complete: we can better understand whether or not the group-specific treatment efficacy is related to the gradient of prognosis β_1.

As a side issue, it is important to understand that the formulation of a predictive tree as in equation 2 is only a rewriting of the classical main effects models plus treatment-by-covariate interaction, i.e.:

$$\text{logit}(p) = \beta_0 + \beta_1 X + \beta_2 Z + (\beta_3 - \beta_2) Z \cdot X \qquad (3)$$

Once a prognostic tree is built on the control arm, it can be used in the whole sample to understand whether or not treatment effect modifiers are present. To this purpose, however, rather than building a simple prognostic tree classifier, a direct approach relying on tree-based regression for treatment interaction detection is preferable (predictive trees) whenever emphasis is to be given to treatment effect modifiers rather than prognosis. But, as highlighted before, it is always preferable to have the entire tree structure represented by one single equation (2) which contains coefficients both for prognosis and treatment response as in the case of RECPAM method [12].

SIDES, the partitioning method recently proposed by Lipkovich et al. [10, 11], represents a very clear and thorough attempt to identify specific subgroups of responders to treatment.

Unfortunately, the asymmetrical nature of partitioning methods is overshadowed by the urge to identify the ideal subgroup with the highest treatment efficacy. It is of paramount interest, in our view, to keep the entire set of subgroups identified, even those where treatment effects are weaker than expected. Focusing only on the *interesting* parts of the covariates' space is preferable only if we wish to partition a sample that contains a mixed population (i.e. nonresponders or a low treatment efficacy subgroup are present) with the purpose of tailoring a population for future studies.

However, in a phase III trial, as well as in real practice, we are simultaneously interested in both types of subgroups: those who responded to treatment and those who did not. Moreover, by simply restricting the interest to the subgroups which most benefit, we might not understand why a generalization of trial results is not possible. And we could miss as well the key feature of deriving an evidence-based treatment algorithm, especially when more than two treatments are at issue (see 'Applications and Extensions of Tree-Based Methods in Neurological Disorders').

Nonetheless, the SIDES method should be acknowledged as one the most innovative and flexible approaches from a clinical standpoint since the authors have proven how clinical stability in prediction and modeling benefits preselection of the candidate covariates based on variable importance derived from a preliminary random forest [11], and enriched traditional methods of partitioning with extra features whose nature is more oriented to clinical meaningfulness than statistical significance [10].

As for GUIDE, the key features are many and the paradigm is extremely flexible. The end point can be binary, multinomial, time to event, or counts. Longitudinal trees and quantile regression are also allowed. Its major characteristic is that the algorithm yields unbiased splits, i.e. the approach corrects for the unequal chance for a covariate to be selected according to whether it is continuous, ordinal, or categorical.

Benchmarking Tree-Based Model Performance and Assessment of Prediction Ability with the Novel Reclassification Measures

Tree-based methods can be preferable to standard main effects modeling because their representation is clinically intuitive and often more appealing. Nonetheless, tree model performance needs to be comparatively assessed against common methods of analysis according to some measures of performance. A brief outline is provided here.

Referring for sake of simplicity to binary outcomes or their extension to time-to-event models, we can argue that a clinical model is good when the individuals experiencing the end point have a higher probability for the event itself if compared to individuals who do not experience the event.

In terms of discrimination ability, the geometrical area under a receiver operating characteristic curve (AUC-ROC) is a well-established measure which contrasts false-positive and true-positive rates according to different cutoff points for predictive probability of the outcome. Its equivalent measure is called the c-index. An AUC-ROC equal to 1 means perfect classification or prediction, while the lower extreme of 0.5 corresponds to classification by chance. AUC-ROC, by the way, reflects poor sensitivity to the inclusion of a new predictor within a reference model [13], which in a tree corresponds somehow to undetectable sensitivity for an added split.

A further common criterion to define a predictive model's accuracy is calibration, which assesses the agreement between observed and predicted proportion of events [13]. We will not discuss calibration for tree algorithms here as, for them, alternative approaches are necessary and would go far beyond the scope of this chapter.

Model performance and prediction ability can be evaluated according to the novel reclassification measures developed by Pencina and

Table 1. Discrimination, calibration, and reclassification measures for event risk prediction at 1 year in ALS patients adding the continuous and the categorical SNIP variable into a reference clinical based model

Model	Survival c-statistic (95% CI)	p value (survival c-statistic difference)	p value (model's Calibration)	cNRI	cNRI events	cNRI-non-events	p value (cNRI)
CEPM[1]	0.839 (0.708–0.971)						
CEPM + SNIP (cont)[2]	0.907 (0.850–0.963)	0.069	0.996	0.582	0.310	0.272	0.036
CEPM + SNIP (tree-str)[3]	0.911 (0.847–0.974)	0.062	0.903	0.771	0.352	0.419	0.009

CEPM = Clinical Established Prediction Model. [1] Included age, sex, BMI, Charlson Comorbidity Index, Amyotrophic Lateral Sclerosis Functional Rating Scale revisited, forced vital capacity, site of onset, and disease duration. [2] Included SNIP as a continuous variable. [3] Included SNIP as a categorical variable, with categories defined from results of RECPAM analysis. SNIP was categorized into the following three classes: class 1 = SNIP $\leq$18 cmH$_2$O; class 2 = 18 < SNIP $\leq$51 cmH$_2$O; class 3 = SNIP >51 cmH$_2$O.

colleagues [14]. These new measures can straightforwardly take into account the interaction between covariates by assessing the added value of each single covariate or split in the tree-building sequence of the partitioning algorithm. They have recently received a lot of attention as these indices intuitively focus on what, for example, a new marker can actually add to a clinically established prediction model. Their names are Integrated Discrimination Improvement (IDI) and Net Reclassification Improvement (NRI), and they both assess, in a straightforward fashion based on predicted probabilities derived from the models compared, the contribution of the added predictor in correctly reclassifying what has been wrongly classified before [13, 14].

In table 1 we show that these novel statistical measures [in this case the continuous version of NRI (cNRI)] provide alternative clinical information if compared to classical measures of model performance [15]. The cNRIs reported represent the relative amount of events and nonevents correctly reclassified by adding a predictor. In this study, 100 ALS patients were enrolled between 2006 and 2010. A tree-structured Cox regression analysis based on the RECPAM algorithm [12] was used to identify subgroups at different risks

for tracheostomy or death. When added to a multivariate clinical established prediction model, the Sniff Nasal Inspiratory Pressure (SNIP) test correctly reclassified the risk of the composite event within 1 year of follow-up. Instead of using SNIP as a continuous variable, the authors were interested in detecting and validating possible cutoffs. Therefore, it was necessary to yield reliable measures of performance for the prediction model. Table 1 clearly reflects the model building strategy and how cNRI for events and nonevents confirmed the superiority of the RECPAM tree-based approach which had selected SNIP as a categorical prognostic factor in three classes. Indeed, this study showed that SNIP measurement in the early phase of the disease may contribute to identify patients with high risk of mortality or intubation, and that could be an additional tool for baseline stratification of patients with ALS in clinical trials.

Notwithstanding the intuitive appealing formulation of cNRI and IDI, some controversies have appeared in the literature and important caveats have been proposed against possible misuse of them. A thorough review and a guide for researchers has recently been published [14]. To this purpose, in the study by Capozzo et al. [15], the improvements in prediction ability provided by the tree-structured cutoffs for SNIP were confirmed by a sensitivity analysis (see Appendix material in [15]) which assessed cNRI within a time horizon from 1 to 3 years and with arbitrarily small positive quantities greater than zero for differences in models' predictive values.

Applications and Extensions of Tree-Based Methods in Neurological Disorders

In the wake of the renewed attention, trees are mainly applied in targeting populations for new trials and in stratified medicine, whose extent, according to many, is expected to be revolutionary.

Subgroups of patients can be identified, for instance, in the early phase of a trial, and eventually tested in a sort of adaptive design fashion. However, the most common application of tree-growing algorithms is their retrospective use to analyze clinical trials who failed to prove overall efficacy and where preplanned subgroup analyses might as well have missed the chance to detect any statistically significant treatment effect.

In our view, a broader vision of the potential strengths of tree algorithms can take us even farther. Their actual vantage point must not be underestimated. Some extensions are provided here.

A tree structure is the natural framework to understand and derive an evidence-based treatment algorithm, especially when we are dealing with more than one treatment, e.g. in a pooled sample of individual patients' data coming from different phase III placebo-controlled trials. This scenario practically corresponds to a subgroup analysis for a mixed treatment comparisons or network meta-analysis [16] driven by a partitioning method algorithm. Formally, wherever possible, we could also perform subgroup-specific head-to-head comparisons.

It should be noted that prior caution is necessary when dealing with pooled data in a mixed treatment comparisons fashion, as all the concerns and caveats of indirect comparison must be taken into account: completeness of the network geometry, statistical and conceptual heterogeneity, and possible incoherence [16].

Subgroup analyses within a network meta-analysis of individual patient data driven by a tree-based algorithm, though they appear a quite straightforward and clinically intuitive question, represent a challenging area of methodological research. The state of the art of tree-growing methods still needs to provide a theoretically sound extension to splitting functions for predictive trees which deal with multiple unordered treatments and appropriately account for heterogeneity between studies. In the absence of a general criterion for the splitting rule, the only viable option now for multiple unordered treatments is to assume the pooled control arms as the reference category for the splitting function, maximizing heterogeneity of effect in all the treatments. This is, of course, a reasonable assumption only if the event rate in the control arms from different trials is not heterogeneous. The process of partitioning itself, however, can be an appropriate way to explore heterogeneity between the control arms since, if covariate-dependent, it can be clearly explained in terms of differential prognosis. Moreover, a weak geometry of the network can pose serious concerns on the ability to control for potential between-trials heterogeneity, unless we can inform the network with many trials per specific comparisons.

Overall, challenging questions are often posed to biostatisticians, and it is surprising how much one can borrow from borderline clinical areas of research. Among neurological disorders, the case of multiple sclerosis (MS) is undoubtedly one of the most favorable for the application and extension of tree-growing techniques. In MS, although not directly derived through a tree-based algorithm, clear examples of a tree-shaped prognostic classifier or treatment effect modifiers have been proposed [3, 17, 18] (fig. 2).

The modified Río score is a statistically driven scoring system which captures the interaction

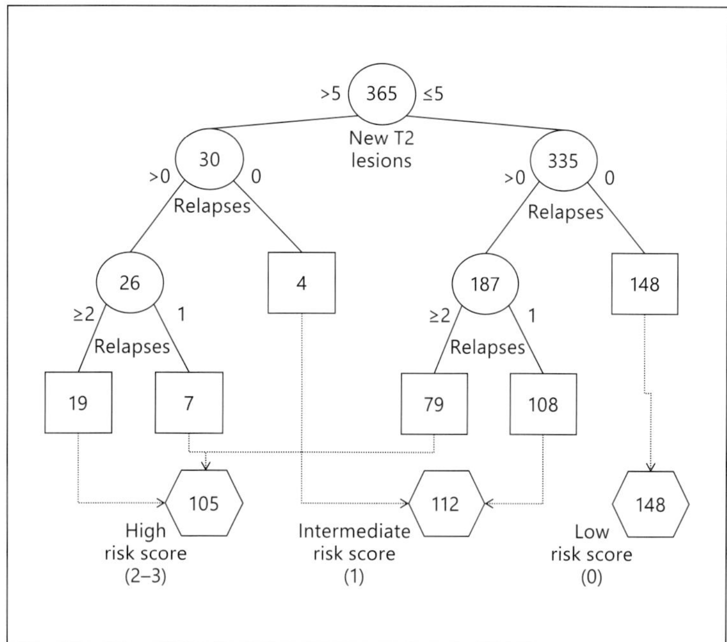

Fig. 2. The modified Río score represented in a tree-structured form. Hexagons represent the amalgamation in three classes or risk score of the six possible strata determined by the interaction between number of relapses (0, 1, ≥2) and new T2 lesions (≤5, >5).

between magnetic resonance imaging and clinical measures (i.e., number of new T2 lesions and relapses at 1 year from baseline assessment) in relapsing remitting MS patients treated with interferon-β in the prediction over 3 years of relapse rates and MS disease progression measured by the Expanded Disability Status Scale (EDSS) (see [17] for specific details). This score system assumes a value from 0 to 3 and is the modification of a previous one [18] in which the prediction of the outcomes was based also on EDSS measured at 1 year from baseline assessment.

Both the original approach by Río et al. [18] and the subsequent modification by Sormani et al. [17] suffer from lack of flexibility in the cutoff points for the predictors used. The Río score dichotomized EDSS, relapses, and new T2 lesions with a priori clinically defined fixed cutoff points to produce eight risk strata (a kind of natural a priori stratification), whereas the modified Río score selected the cutoff points following a naïve algorithm-based process similar to a tree-based

approach, but completely missed the concern of potential bias in the splitting procedure due to the unequal chance of being selected dictated by the continuous, ordinal, or categorical nature of the covariates as detailed for the GUIDE approach at the end of 'Prognosis and Treatment-by-Covariate Interactions via Tree-Based Methods'.

Besides, in the modified Río score, EDSS is a priori dismissed from the set of prognostic factors, relying on the assumption that surrogacy has been proven between the relapse rate and EDSS, and therefore that relapses only could be included in the model for predicting treatment response. As a side concern, since no control arm has actually been used in its application so far [3], it would be misleading to talk of treatment response in the strict sense of an effect modifier.

The tree-shaped modified Río score displayed in figure 2 shows the covariate new T2 lesions as the most important split, below which further splits for relapses occur. It is straightforward to understand that an equivalent representation could have been obtained placing relapses on the top of the tree and then splitting further for new T2 lesions. We would obtain the same six combinations of leaves.

In contrast, a tree-based approach would directly derive and establish a hierarchy of importance of the covariates to define the new scoring system, and, most remarkably, unbiased cutoffs would be determined and cross-validated by the algorithm while taking into account the role of concurring baseline covariates by adding them either in the reference model as global predictors [12] or allowing them to be potentially selected in the tree structure. Moreover, EDSS could and should be reintroduced and directly tested to understand whether and when it is selected by the tree algorithm.

A future extension on this topic consists of exploring the prognostic nature versus the predictive nature of the modified Río score applied to a pooled sample of phase III placebo-controlled trials regarding interferon-β and other disease-modifying therapies for MS. It would be interesting to understand, for instance, whether or not cutoffs for the components of the score are drug-specific.

In general, we should make clear that, as trees are a well-grounded overall strategy for building prediction models, it is also very important to rely on powerful statistical tools especially when covariate-treatment interactions are at issue. Tree-structured regression and its extension to an ensemble of trees [7–12] are suitable statistical models. Particularly, ensembles of trees, also known as random forests [8, 11], though losing some intuitive appeal in the interpretation of the interactions when compared to regression trees, extend the predictive ability to higher levels and easily allow stability and internal validation via bootstrap or cross-validation techniques, especially when the number of covariates (i.e. potential genetic or clinical biomarkers and risk factors) is much greater than the number of subjects.

Further advances correspond to extend tree-growing techniques to real-life data sources. By accounting for the clustered nature of some designs (e.g. multicenter observational studies), we would be able to address the role of the prescribers and whether or how they influence an evidence-based treatment algorithm derived in a randomized clinical trial framework. However, in this case, methods to overcome the absence of randomization are necessary. To this purpose, a tree-based regression integrating propensity score methods has been proposed [19, 20].

Last, tree-growing techniques can be used to address a posteriori subgroups analyses to understand why a phase III trial did not show efficacy, as well as to tailor in terms of treatment response a target population for new trials. When addressing prognostic stratification only, trees are the ideal statistical framework to select and validate the most appropriate combination of covariates and cutoffs, as in the case of the reassessment of the Río and modified Río scores. Additionally, as discussed in 'Benchmarking Tree-Based Model Performance and Assessment of Prediction Ability with the Novel Reclassification Measures', it is important to benchmark model performance and to assess the added value of specific covariates according to (survival) c-index, integrated discrimination improvement, and continuous net reclassification improvement.

References

1 Mitsumoto H, Brooks BR, Silani V: Clinical trials in amyotrophic lateral sclerosis: why so many negative trials and how can trials be improved? Lancet Neurol 2014;13:1127–1138.

2 Matthews PM, Edison P, Geraghty OC, Johnson MR: The emerging agenda of stratified medicine in neurology. Nat Rev Neurol 2014;10:15–26.

3 Sormani MP, De Stefano N: Defining and scoring response to IFN-β in multiple sclerosis. Nat Rev Neurol 2013;9:504–512.

4 Janes H, Pepe MS, Huang Y: A framework for evaluating markers used to select patient treatment. Med Decis Making 2014;34:159–167.

5 Zhao L, Tian L, Cai T, Claggett B, Wei LJ: Effectively selecting a target population for a future comparative study. J Am Stat Assoc 2013;108:527–539.

6 Piepho HP, Madden LV, Williams ER: Multiplicative interaction in network meta-analysis. Stat Med 2014;34:582–594.

7 Loh WY, He X, Man M: A regression tree approach to identifying subgroups with differential treatment effects. Stat Med 2015;34:1818–1833.

8 Loh WY: Classification and regression trees, WIREsData Mining Knowl Discov 2011;1:14–23.

9 Loh WY: Fifty years of classification and regression trees (with discussion). Int Stat Rev 2014;34:329–370.

10 Lipkovich I, Dmitrienko A, Denne J, Enas G: Subgroup identification based on differential effect search: a recursive partitioning method for establishing response to treatment in patient subpopulations. Stat Med 2011;30:2601–2621.

11 Lipkovich I, Dmitrienko A: Strategies for identifying predictive biomarkers and subgroups with enhanced treatment effect in clinical trials using SIDES. J Biopharm Stat 2014;24:130–153.

12 Ciampi A, Negassa A, Lou Z: Tree-structured prediction for censored survival data and the Cox model. J Clin Epidemiol 1995;48:675–689.

13 Cook NR: Use and misuse of the receiver operating characteristic curve in risk prediction. Circulation 2007;115:928–935.

14 Leening MJ, Vedder MM, Witteman JC, Pencina MJ, Steyerberg EW: Net reclassification improvement: computation, interpretation, and controversies: a literature review and clinician's guide. Ann Intern Med 2014;160:122–131.

15 Capozzo R, Quaranta VN, Pellegrini F, et al: Sniff nasal inspiratory pressure as a prognostic factor of tracheostomy or death in amyotrophic lateral sclerosis. J Neurol 2015;262:593–603.

16 Mills EJ, Thorlund K, Ioannidis JP: Demystifying trial networks and network meta-analysis. BMJ 2013;346:f2914.

17 Sormani MP, Rio J, Tintorè M, et al: Scoring treatment response in patients with relapsing multiple sclerosis. Mult Scler 2013;19:605–612.

18 Río J, Nos C, Tintoré M, et al: Defining the response to interferon-beta in relapsing-remitting multiple sclerosis patients. Ann Neurol 2006;59:344–352.

19 Kang J, Su X, Hitsman B, Liu K, Lloyd-Jones D: Tree-structured analysis of treatment effects with large observational data. J Appl Stat 2012;39:513–529.

20 Su X, Kang J, Fan J, Levine RA, Yan X: Facilitating score and causal inference trees for large observational studies. J Mach Learn Res 2012;13:2955–2994.

Massimiliano Copetti, PhD
Unit of Biostatistics, IRCCS Casa Sollievo della Sofferenza
Viale Padre Pio
IT–71013 San Giovanni Rotondo (Italy)
E-Mail m.copetti@operapadrepio.it

Beghi E, Logroscino G (eds): The Right Therapy for Neurological Disorders. From Randomized Trials to Clinical Practice.
Front Neurol Neurosci. Basel, Karger, 2016, vol 39, pp 60–70 (DOI: 10.1159/000445413)

Composite Scores and Other Outcome Measures in Stroke Trials

Francesca Pistoia · Simona Sacco · Raffaele Ornello · Diana Degan · Cindy Tiseo · Antonio Carolei

Neurological Institute, Department of Biotechnological and Applied Clinical Sciences, University of L'Aquila, L'Aquila, Italy

Abstract

Background: Randomized controlled trials represent the most useful tool to evaluate the effectiveness of a treatment in medical research. When designing a clinical trial, the choice of end points, assessment tools, and scores is crucial as they represent the prerequisites for the evaluation of outcomes and for the critical appraisal of findings. ***Summary:*** In stroke research, outcomes are mainly represented by composite end points focusing on the occurrence of cardiovascular and cerebrovascular events in trials on primary and secondary prevention and by measures of recovery and residual disability in acute stroke trials. Assessment tools which are more frequently used to evaluate recovery after acute stroke care include the National Institutes of Health Stroke Scale, the Modified Rankin Scale, the Barthel Index, the Glasgow Outcome Scale, and the Stroke Impact Scale. However, there is a wide heterogeneity of outcome measures across different trials, which makes it difficult to compare results and to draw definitive conclusions on the usefulness of the investigated strategies and treatments. Moreover, in some cases, details about outcomes are poorly reported with a tendency to focus on outcomes that are statistically significant while information about nonsignificant outcomes is frequently missed. ***Key Messages:*** There is an urgent need to improve the quality of designing, conducting, analyzing, and reporting data from randomized clinical trials in order to obtain complete, clear, and rigorous information on the effectiveness of management strategies in stroke care. Key properties of tools measuring outcome should include validity, reliability, and convenient statistical characteristics. © 2016 S. Karger AG, Basel

A wide range of outcome measures may be adopted in stroke trials to estimate outcomes and quality of life after a stroke. Outcome measures differ across various trials: they are mainly represented by composite end points focusing on the occurrence of cardiovascular and cerebrovascular events in trials on primary and secondary prevention of stroke and by measures of residual disability in trials investigating the effects of acute stroke treatments. The former quantify to what extent primary and secondary prevention strategies are able to reduce the incidence of first-ever and recurrent strokes, whereas the latter evaluate recovery and quality of life of patients who have experienced a stroke. Such outcome measures are often too heterogeneous across different trials and do not allow reliable comparisons to be made among the investigated groups.

Outcomes in Trials on Primary and Secondary Prevention of Stroke

Trials on primary and secondary prevention of stroke are extremely numerous and heterogeneous, especially with respect to the investigated outcomes. The aims of these trials have been to investigate the usefulness of lifestyle strategies as well as the effectiveness of various treatments, including blood pressure lowering drugs, antidiabetic and cholesterol/triglyceride-lowering medications, and antiplatelet or anticoagulant drugs in the prevention of first-ever or recurrent strokes. The findings of these trials represent the starting point to draw up international recommendations and guidelines for the proper prevention of stroke [1, 2]. A considerable number of trials have been focused on the effectiveness of blood-pressure-lowering drugs as preventive agents for stroke [3]. Primary and secondary end points are usually represented by composite outcomes addressing the occurrence of cardiovascular and cerebrovascular events. A comprehensive meta-analysis of these trials recently identified 147 studies, including 108 blood pressure difference trials investigating blood pressure differences between study drugs and placebo, and 46 drug comparison trials comparing the effects of different drugs [4]. Within the former, the number of incident strokes was reported by the majority of trials, although stroke was reported as an independent outcome only in 13 studies [4]. Within the latter, stroke was reported as the primary outcome in 4 studies and as a secondary outcome in another 4 trials; the remaining studies did not establish any hierarchy among outcome events [4]. Another meta-analysis included 24 randomized trials that compared the effects of the six major blood-pressure-lower-

ing drugs: stroke was reported in all trials as either the primary or secondary outcome, although the definition of stroke varied among the different studies [5]. In most of those trials, primary and secondary end points were usually composite. For instance, in the Heart Outcomes Prevention Evaluation (HOPE) Study, the primary outcome was a composite of myocardial infarction, stroke, or death from cardiovascular causes [6]. Similarly, in the Telmisartan Randomised Assessment Study in ACE Intolerant Subjects with Cardiovascular Disease (TRANSCEND), the primary outcome was the composite of cardiovascular death, myocardial infarction, stroke, or hospitalization for heart failure [7]. In the Morbidity and Mortality after Stroke, Eprosartan Compared with Nitrendipine for Secondary Prevention (MOSES) study, the primary end point was a composite of total mortality and all cardiovascular and cerebrovascular events including all recurring events [8], while in the Valsartan Antihypertensive Long-Term Use Evaluation (VALUE) study, fatal and nonfatal stroke was part of the secondary end points together with fatal and nonfatal myocardial infarction and fatal and nonfatal heart failure [9]. Stroke belonged to composite secondary end points also in the Ongoing Telmisartan Alone and in Combination with Ramipril Global Endpoint Trial (ONTARGET) where a composite of death from cardiovascular causes, myocardial infarction, or stroke was analyzed [10]. On the other hand, stroke was investigated as a secondary independent outcome in the Anglo-Scandinavian Cardiac Outcomes Trial-Blood Pressure Lowering Arm (ASCOT-BPLA), while the primary end point was a composite of nonfatal myocardial infarction and fatal coronary heart disease [11]. Finally, the recent Systolic Blood Pressure Intervention Trial (SPRINT), which investigated whether intensive blood pressure control aimed at obtaining blood pressure targets of less than 120 mm Hg is better than the standard control in the prevention of cardiovascular and cerebrovascular diseases, considered the occurrence of stroke as a part of a primary composite outcome also including myocardial infarction, other acute coronary syndromes, heart failure, or death from cardiovascular causes [12].

In primary prevention trials investigating the effects of cholesterol-/triglyceride-lowering drugs, the occurrence of stroke was considered as either a primary or a secondary outcome. In the Justification for the Use of Statins in Primary Prevention: An Intervention Trial Evaluating Rosuvastatin (JUPITER), stroke was included in the composite primary outcome together with nonfatal myocardial infarction, hospitalization for unstable angina, arterial revascularization procedure, and confirmed death from cardiovascular causes [13]. With respect to secondary prevention, fatal or nonfatal stroke was investigated as the primary outcome in the Stroke Prevention by Aggressive Reduction in Cholesterol Levels (SPARCL) trial [14]. On the other hand, stroke was considered as a secondary outcome in the Long-Term Intervention with Pravastatin in Ischemic Disease (LIPID) trial [15], the Antihypertensive and Lipid-Lowering Treatment to Prevent Heart Attack Trial (ALLHAT) [16], the Heart Protection Study (HPS) [17], the Anglo-Scandinavian Cardiac Outcomes Trial-Lipid Lowering Arm (ASCOT-LLA) trial [18], and the Primary Prevention of Cardiovascular Disease with Pravastatin in Japan (MEGA) Study [19].

As regards the management of diabetes mellitus, a recent meta-analysis addressed the effects of an intensive control of glucose on the incidence of stroke [20]: stroke was reported as an independent outcome in the Diabetes Insulin-Glucose in Acute Myocardial Infarction (DIGAMI) and in the UK Prospective Diabetes Study (UKPDS) Group trials, while it was investigated in the framework of a composite primary outcome in the Nateglinide + Valsartan to Prevent or Delay Type II Diabetes Mellitus and Cardiovascular Complications (NAVIGATOR), the Veterans Affairs Diabetes Trial (VADT), the Outcome Reduction with Initial Glargine Intervention (ORIGIN), the Action to Control Cardiovascular Risk in Diabetes

(ACCORD), the Action in Diabetes and Vascular Disease (ADVANCE), and the Prospective Pioglitazone Clinical Trial in Macrovascular Events (PROactive) [20]. Stroke was also investigated independently among secondary outcomes in the three last trials mentioned above [20]. Finally, the recent Insulin Resistance Intervention after Stroke (IRIS) trial investigated the effectiveness of pioglitazone, an insulin-sensitizing drug of the thiazolidinedione class, in reducing the risk of stroke and myocardial infarction among insulin-resistant, nondiabetic patients with a recent ischemic stroke or transient ischemic attack: in this study the primary outcome was time to stroke or myocardial infarction, while secondary outcomes included time to stroke alone, acute coronary syndrome, diabetes, cognitive decline, and all-cause mortality [21]. Differently from what was reported in the aforementioned studies, almost all trials focusing on the effects of antithrombotic drugs investigated the occurrence of ischemic stroke as a primary outcome.

Among trials on the primary prevention of cardiovascular events with acetylsalicylic acid, stroke was considered as an independent primary outcome in the Womens' Health Study [22], the British Doctors' Study [23], and the Physicians' Health Study [24], while it was a part of a composite outcome in the Japanese Primary Prevention of Atherosclerosis with Aspirin for Diabetes (JPAD) trial [25], in the Prevention of Progression of Arterial Disease and Diabetes (POPADAD) trial [26], and in the Aspirin for Asymptomatic Atherosclerosis Trial (AAAT) study [27]. Finally, stroke was investigated as an independent secondary outcome in the JPAD trial [25], in the Thrombosis Prevention Trial (TPT) [28], and in the Hypertension Optimal Treatment (HOT) trial [29].

Among trials investigating the effects of antiplatelet agents in the secondary prevention of stroke, recurrent stroke was investigated as an independent outcome in the Clopidogrel versus Aspirin in Patients at Risk of Ischemic Events trial

[30], the European Stroke Prevention Study 2 [31], the Fast Assessment of Stroke and Transient Ischemic Attack to Prevent Early Recurrence (FASTER) study [32], the Prevention Regimen for Effectively Avoiding Second Strokes (PRoFESS) trial [33], and the Clopidogrel in High-Risk Patients with Acute Nondisabling Cerebrovascular Events (CHANCE) trial [34], while it was reported as belonging to a composite primary outcome including other vascular events in the Aspirin and Clopidogrel Compared with Clopidogrel Alone after Recent Ischaemic Stroke or Transient Ischaemic Attack in High-Risk Patients (MATCH) trial [35], the Clopidogrel for High Atherothrombotic Risk and Ischemic Stabilization, Management, and Avoidance (CHARISMA) trial [36], and in the European/Australasian Stroke Prevention in Reversible Ischaemia (ESPRIT) trial [37]. In trials addressing the effects of both warfarin [38] and direct oral anticoagulants [39–43], stroke was commonly included in composite outcomes. In the Randomized Evaluation of Long-Term Anticoagulation Therapy (RE-LY) trial, stroke was considered independently among secondary outcomes [39]. As regards the secondary prevention of stroke in patients with atrial fibrillation, stroke belonged to a composite primary outcome also including death from vascular disease, myocardial infarction, or systemic embolism in the European Atrial Fibrillation Trial (EAFT) [44], while it was an independent outcome in the Heparin in Acute Embolic Stroke Trial (HAEST) [45].

In trials investigating the benefits arising from the endarterectomy procedure in asymptomatic carotid stenosis, such as the Asymptomatic Carotid Atherosclerosis Study (ACAS) [46], the Asymptomatic Carotid Surgery Trial (ACST) [47], the Veterans Administration Cooperative Study [48], the Stenting and Angioplasty with Protection In Patients at High Risk for Endarterectomy (SAPPHIRE) trial [49], the Carotid Revascularization Endarterectomy versus Stenting Trial (CREST) [50], and the ongoing CREST-2 (ClinicalTrials.gov Identifier: NCT02089217), stroke was usually reported as a primary outcome, albeit with some differences in the used definitions. Recurrent stroke was reported as a primary outcome also in trials investigating the effects of carotid endarterectomy for stroke secondary prevention such as the European Carotid Surgery Trial (ECST) [51], the North American Symptomatic Carotid Endarterectomy Trial (NASCET) [52], and the Veterans Affairs Cooperative Studies Program (VACSP) trial [53]. In addition, in trials comparing the effects of carotid endarterectomy with those of stenting for the secondary prevention of stroke, stroke was commonly reported as a part of composite primary outcomes [54–57]. Finally, among trials for the management of intracranial stenosis in patients with cerebrovascular events, including the Warfarin-Aspirin Symptomatic Intracranial Disease (WASID) trial and the Stenting versus Aggressive Medical Therapy for Intracranial Arterial Stenosis (SAMMPRIS) trial, stroke belonged to a composite primary outcome while it was independently investigated as a secondary outcome [58, 59].

Outcome Measures in Acute Stroke Trials

Recently, the WHO International Classification of Functioning, Disability and Health (ICF) proposed to describe postinjury disability with respect to three different domains: physical impairment, functional activity (formerly disability), or social participation (formerly handicap) [60]. This was an attempt to encourage the use of a common language among researchers and health care professionals and to refer to disability as a multifaceted entity implying an interaction between features of the person and features of the overall context in which the person lives. Within this theoretical framework, the disability rate of an individual is not only the result of the disease-related functional impairment, but also the consequence of the effects of any environmental

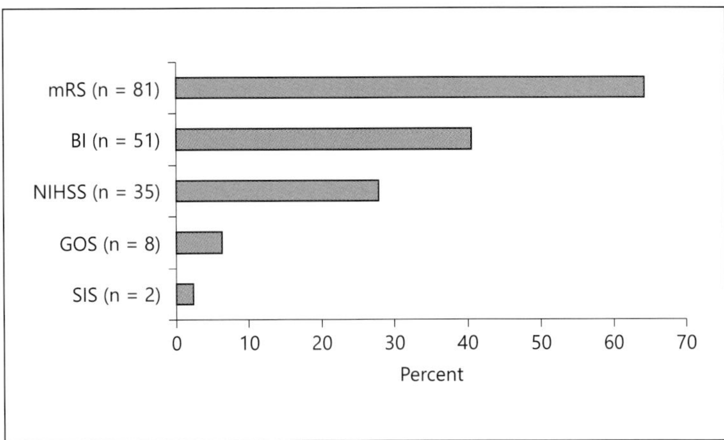

Fig. 1. Number of contemporary stroke trials using main functional outcomes assessment scales (data from [62]).

barriers and facilitators which influence his daily living performances. As a consequence, multiple assessment tools are necessary to evaluate the different domains of postinjury disability and to quantify the effectiveness of any medical and social interventions to reduce its burden. In this respect, the most common outcome measures in stroke trials include the Modified Rankin Scale (mRS), the National Institutes of Health Stroke Scale (NIHSS), the Barthel Index (BI), the Glasgow Outcome Scale (GOS), and the Stroke Impact Scale (SIS) [61].

The mRS is a hierarchical ordinal scale measuring the degree of disability and dependence in daily life activities: the score ranges from 0 to 6, with 0 indicating no symptoms and 6 indicating death. The NIHSS is mainly a measure of neurological impairment: it is a 15-item scale quantifying deficits at the level of consciousness, language, neglect, visual field loss, extraocular movement, motor strength, ataxia, dysarthria, and sensory loss, with an overall score ranging from 0 (no deficit) to 42 (maximal deficit). The BI quantifies the level of performance in 10 basic activities of daily living (feeding, bathing, grooming, dressing, bowel and bladder function, toilet use) and mobility (transfers, mobility on level surfaces and stairs), with a total score ranging from 0 to 100, where the highest scores indicate the greatest independence. The

GOS is a hierarchical ordinal scale scored from 1 (death) to 5 (good recovery). It is also available in an extended version, including eight levels which more deeply stratify levels of disability. The SIS quantifies the magnitude of physical, cognitive, and mood dysfunctions in patients with stroke as well as their residual ability to perform basic daily activities and participate in social activities. The total score ranges from 0 to 100, with 0 representing no recovery and 100 representing full recovery.

Other assessment tools which are only rarely used in acute stroke trials include the Scandinavian Stroke Scale, the EuroQOL, the Frenchay Activities Index, the Timed Walk/6-min Walk, the Functional Independence Measure Scale, the Fugl-Meyer Motor Scale, the Wolf Motor Functional Test, the Rivermead Mobility Index, the Short-Form 36, the Berg Balance Scale, the Canadian Stroke Scale, and the Tinetti Balance Assessment Tool [61, 62]. The frequency of use of the main functional outcomes assessment scales in contemporary stroke trials is shown in figure 1. In addition, most of the acute stroke trials also include neuroimaging outcomes addressing measures of infarct volume, degree of recanalization, mismatch profiles, and percentages of rescued penumbra.

In recent years much attention has been paid to identifying the factors which influence the performance of outcome measures [61]. Desirable properties of stroke outcome measures should include reliability, validity, responsiveness, convenient statistical characteristics, availability of training, cultural and language issues, and resistance to comorbidity [61, 63]. Reliability is an index of whether or not a scale consistently and reproducibly measures the attributes it wants to measure. Test-retest reliability is a measure of the consistency of results over time in the absence of changes in the subject population and the raters, while interrater reliability evaluates the consistency of results among different raters [64]. Test-retest reliability of the mRS has been reported to be strong in various studies (kappa = 0.81–0.95), while interrater reliability of the mRS seems to be moderate and improves with structured interviews (kappa 0.56 versus 0.78) [65]. Test-retest reliability for the NIHSS was also found to be high (kappa = 0.66–0.77) as well as interrater reliability (kappa = 0.69) [66, 67]. Moreover, to further improve the reliability of the NIHSS, a modified version, obtained by excluding NIHSS items with low kappa values, has been recently developed [68]. The reliability of the BI in stroke research is also acceptable as shown by several studies reporting a reliability ranging from moderate (kappa = 0.41–0.60) to good (kappa = 0.61–0.80) to very good (kappa = 0.81–1.00) [69]. The validity of the BI has also been reported to be moderate as confirmed by the association between BI scores and other clinical data, such as the amount of nursing time required by patients, the extent of motor loss, and the size of the infarct [69]. Similarly, a close correlation between BI scores and other measures of activity has been shown [69].

Validity is the degree to which an instrument measures the concept it was intended to measure. Construct validity is measured by using correlation coefficients to test a newly developed scale against a previously used scale while convergent validity shows whether a test is correlated with other tests designed to measure theoretically similar concepts [64]. Several studies have endorsed the construct validity of the mRS by reporting that location, type, and extent of stroke injury are closely related to short- and longer-term disability as quantified by the mRS [65], whereas others have documented the convergent validity between the mRS and other disability scales [70, 71]. The validity of the NIHSS was also acceptable as endorsed by a good correlation between the scale scores of patients and the patients' infarction size (r = 0.68) and the patients' clinical outcome as determined at 3 months (r = 0.79) [71]. The modified version of the NIHSS has been reported to have a high validity as the original NIHSS [68].

Less data are available about the reliability and validity of the GOS and the SIS. However, the GOS correlates with the mRS in most patients with stroke, showing a good concurrent validity, while the SIS has been reported to have a high intrarater reliability (intraclass correlations ranging from 0.7 to 0.92) and a good-to-excellent concurrent validity [72].

As shown by data from the Virtual International Stroke Trials Archive (VISTA), there is a strong correlation among NIHSS, mRS, and BI scores across different studies (Spearman's rho coefficient between 3-month mRS and BI: –0.94; Spearman's rho coefficient between 3-month mRS and NIHSS score: 0.91; Spearman's rho coefficient between NIHSS and BI: –0.85) [61, 73]. By analyzing the distribution of the different scores within the investigated populations in stroke trials, it is also evident that BI may suffer from floor and ceiling effects, with a slight variation of scores at the lower and upper ends of the potential range, whereas NIHSS may be affected by a ceiling effect alone [61]. Some studies also investigated the correlation between clinical and neuroimaging outcomes in stroke trials. In this respect, a substudy of the Randomized Trial of Tirilazad Mesylate in Patients with Acute Stroke (RANTTAS) investigated the correlation between the infarct volume and location, assessed by computed tomography scan on 6–11 days following the acute event, and the 3-month outcome assessed by means of

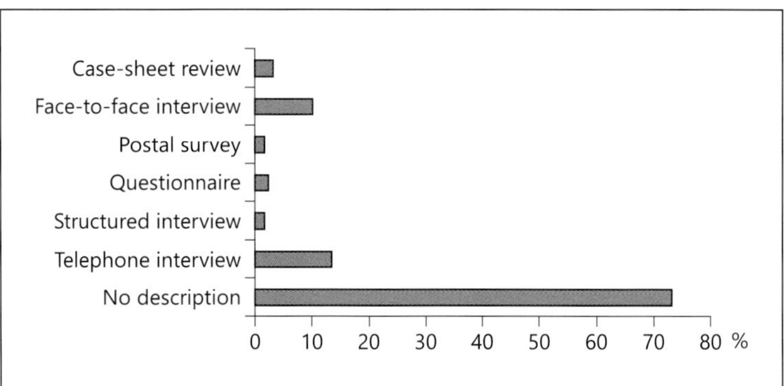

Fig. 2. Frequency of use of different assessment methodologies for stroke functional outcomes across contemporary stroke trials (data from [62]).

NIHSS, BI, and GOS tools, and reported a moderate correlation between neuroimaging and clinical outcomes (Spearman's rho coefficient between infarct volume and NIHSS: 0.54; Spearman's rho coefficient between infarct volume and BI: 0.43; Spearman's rho coefficient between infarct volume and GOS: 0.53) [74]. A more recent study found a significant correlation between the decreased apparent diffusion coefficient value on diffusion-weighted magnetic resonance imaging of patients with acute stroke and the 6-month outcome assessed with GOS (r = 0.73), mRS (r = 0.68), and BI (r = 0.67) [75]. Finally, other studies have evaluated the correlation between the perfusion-diffusion mismatch profile, as a surrogate of the ischemic penumbra, and the clinical outcomes of patients [76, 77].

Heterogeneity of Outcomes and Assessment Methodologies in Stroke Research

The availability of such numerous assessment tools make the findings of different clinical trials extremely heterogeneous and make it difficult to compare them and draw definite conclusions. This heterogeneity is mainly from the wide number of physical and psychological domains which may be affected after a stroke. Some assessment tools mainly focus on neurological impairment and on the loss of specific skills, while others provide information about the degree of functional independence in daily living and the presence of environmental factors and barriers which prevent the subject to perform his activities and to meet his own expectations about daily life and social participation. The above heterogeneity is also the result of different timing and assessment modalities across stroke studies as data may be collected at different time intervals following the acute event and through multiple assessment techniques including case-sheet review, face-to-face interview, telephone interview, video recorded interview, postal survey, and the use of structured questionnaires [62]. The frequency of use of different assessment methodologies for stroke functional outcomes is shown in figure 2. Finally, further heterogeneity may arise from differences across the various studies in processing and analyzing the data. In acute stroke trials, for example, it occurs that mRS ordinal categories are dichotomized into a binary outcome denoting a good or a poor outcome. However, the lack of uniformity in the established cutoff points becomes a source of confusion in comparing data from different trials. In the light of these difficulties and in order to make results mutually comparable, future trials should use validated outcome assessment tools, select uniform methods of application and analysis, and provide complete, clear, and transparent information about the adopted methodology. In this respect, the most recent guidelines from the

Consolidated Standards of Reporting Trials (CONSORT) group provided specific recommendations for investigators to encourage clarity, completeness, and transparency in describing a trial's methodology [78]. With respect to outcomes, investigators are recommended to properly describe prespecified primary and secondary outcome measures and to report how and when they were assessed. Moreover, it is recommended that the description of the methodology should include sufficient details to allow replication, and that any changes involving the choice and the estimation of outcomes after the beginning of the trial be clearly reported [78]. Finally, when publishing results from randomized clinical trials, the so-called 'outcome reporting bias', which arises from the widespread tendency to focus on outcomes that are statistically significant while details about nonsignificant outcomes are often omitted, should be avoided [79].

Future Directions

As already reported, the most challenging issue in comparing results from different stroke trials is coping with too many heterogeneous outcome measures. This heterogeneity cannot be renounced as it is the consequence of the composite nature of disability which is influenced by several parameters including body structures, functions, activity, and participation. To overcome this issue, the use of a composite measure, derived from the combination of scores from multiple scales, has been advocated by the National Institute of Neurological Disorders and Stroke (NINDS). An attempt to test a composite measure has been performed in the framework of the NINDS t-PA Stroke Trial, where it has been suggested to define the primary outcome as a 'consistent and persuasive difference' in the proportion of patients achieving favorable outcomes on the BI, mRS, GOS, and NIHSS [80]. The conclusion of the workshop was that a global statistic may be proposed to test the trial's primary hypothesis followed by secondary tests of individual outcomes [80]. However, the acceptance of this approach within the scientific community was not great and global testing has rarely been used in later clinical trials. The gold standard for future clinical trials would be to develop a more comprehensive scale addressing the various aspects of recovery and disability.

References

1 Meschia JF, Bushnell C, Boden-Albala B, et al: Guidelines for the primary prevention of stroke: a statement for healthcare professionals from the American Heart Association/American Stroke Association. Stroke 2014;45:3754–3832.

2 Kernan WN, Ovbiagele B, Black HR, et al: Guidelines for the prevention of stroke in patients with stroke and transient ischemic attack: a guideline for healthcare professionals from the American Heart Association/American Stroke Association. Stroke 2014;45: 2160–2236.

3 Pistoia F, Sacco S, Degan D, Tiseo C, Ornello R, Carolei A: Hypertension and stroke: epidemiological aspects and clinical evaluation. High Blood Press Cardiovasc Prev 2016;23:9–18.

4 Law MR, Morris JK, Wald NJ: Use of blood pressure lowering drugs in the prevention of cardiovascular disease: meta-analysis of 147 randomised trials in the context of expectations from prospective epidemiological studies. BMJ 2009;338:b1665.

5 Wright JM, Musini VM: First-line drugs for hypertension. Cochrane Database Syst Rev 2009;3:CD001841.

6 Yusuf S, Sleight P, Pogue J, Bosch J, Davies R, Dagenais G: Effects of an angiotensin-converting-enzyme inhibitor, ramipril, on cardiovascular events in high-risk patients. The Heart Outcomes Prevention Evaluation Study Investigators. N Engl J Med 2000;342:145–153.

7 Yusuf S, Teo K, Anderson C, et al: Effects of the angiotensin-receptor blocker telmisartan on cardiovascular events in high-risk patients intolerant to angiotensin-converting enzyme inhibitors: a randomised controlled trial. Lancet 2008;372:1174–1183.

8 Schrader J, Lüders S, Kulschewski A, Hammersen F, Plate K, Berger J, Zidek W, Dominiak P, Diener HC; MOSES Study Group: Morbidity and mortality after stroke, eprosartan compared with nitrendipine for secondary prevention: principal results of a prospective randomized controlled study (MOSES). Stroke 2005;36:1218–1226.

9 Julius S, Kjeldsen SE, Weber M, et al: Outcomes in hypertensive patients at high cardiovascular risk treated with regimens based on valsartan or amlodipine: the VALUE randomised trial. Lancet 2004;363:2022–2031.

10 Yusuf S, Teo KK, Pogue J, et al: Telmisartan, ramipril, or both in patients at high risk for vascular events. N Engl J Med 2008;358:1547–1559.

11 Dahlöf B, Sever PS, Poulter NR, et al: Prevention of cardiovascular events with an antihypertensive regimen of amlodipine adding perindopril as required versus atenolol adding bendroflumethiazide as required, in the Anglo-Scandinavian Cardiac Outcomes Trial-Blood Pressure Lowering Arm (ASCOT-BPLA): a multicentre randomised controlled trial. Lancet 2005;366:895–906.

12 The SPRINT Research Group: A randomized trial of intensive versus standard blood-pressure control. N Engl J Med 2015;373:2103–2116.

13 Ridker PM, Danielson E, Fonseca FA, et al: Rosuvastatin to prevent vascular events in men and women with elevated C-reactive protein. N Engl J Med 2008; 359:2195–2207.

14 Amarenco P, Bogousslavsky J, Callahan A 3rd, et al: High-dose atorvastatin after stroke or transient ischemic attack. N Engl J Med 2006;355:549–559.

15 The Long-Term Intervention with Pravastatin in Ischaemic Disease (LIPID) Study Group: Prevention of cardiovascular events and death with pravastatin in patients with coronary heart disease and a broad range of initial cholesterol levels. N Engl J Med 1998;339:1349–1357.

16 ALLHAT Officers and Coordinators for the ALLHAT Collaborative Research Group; the Antihypertensive and Lipid-Lowering Treatment to Prevent Heart Attack Trial: Major outcomes in moderately hypercholesterolemic, hypertensive patients randomized to pravastatin vs usual care: the Antihypertensive and Lipid-Lowering Treatment to Prevent Heart Attack Trial (ALLHAT-LLT). JAMA 2002;288:2998–3007.

17 Heart Protection Study Collaborative Group: MRC/BHF Heart Protection Study of cholesterol lowering with simvastatin in 20,536 high-risk individuals: a randomised placebo-controlled trial. Lancet 2002;360:7–22.

18 Sever PS, Dahlöf B, Poulter NR, et al: Prevention of coronary and stroke events with atorvastatin in hypertensive patients who have average or lower-than-average cholesterol concentrations, in the Anglo-Scandinavian Cardiac Outcomes Trial-Lipid Lowering Arm (ASCOT-LLA): a multicentre randomised controlled trial. Lancet 2003; 361:1149–1158.

19 Nakamura H, Arakawa K, Itakura H, et al: Primary prevention of cardiovascular disease with pravastatin in Japan (MEGA Study): a prospective randomised controlled trial. Lancet 2006; 368:1155–1163.

20 Zhang C, Zhou YH, Xu CL, Chi FL, Ju HN: Efficacy of intensive control of glucose in stroke prevention: a meta-analysis of data from 59,197 participants in 9 randomized controlled trials. PLoS One 2013;8:e54465.

21 Viscoli CM, Brass LM, Carolei A, et al: Pioglitazone for secondary prevention after ischemic stroke and transient ischemic attack: rationale and design of the Insulin Resistance Intervention after Stroke Trial. Am Heart J 2014;168:823–829.e6.

22 Ridker PM, Cook NR, Lee IM, et al: A randomized trial of low-dose aspirin in the primary prevention of cardiovascular disease in women. N Engl J Med 2005;352:1293–1304.

23 Peto R, Gray R, Collins R, et al: Randomised trial of prophylactic daily aspirin in British male doctors. BMJ 1988; 296:313–316.

24 Steering Committee of the Physicians' Health Study Research Group: Final report on the aspirin component of the ongoing Physicians' Health Study. N Engl J Med 1989;321:129–135.

25 Ogawa H, Nakayama M, Morimoto T, et al: Low-dose aspirin for primary prevention of atherosclerotic events in patients with type 2 diabetes: a randomized controlled trial. JAMA 2008;300:2134–2141.

26 Belch J, MacCuish A, Campbell I, et al: The Prevention of Progression of Arterial Disease and Diabetes (POPADAD) trial: factorial randomized placebo controlled trial of aspirin and antioxidants in patients with diabetes and asymptomatic peripheral arterial disease. BMJ 2008;337:a1840.

27 Fowkes FG, Price JF, Stewart MC, et al: Aspirin for prevention of cardiovascular events in a population screened for a low ankle brachial index. JAMA 2010; 303:841–848.

28 Thrombosis Prevention Trial: randomized trial of low intensity oral anticoagulation with warfarin and low-dose aspirin in the primary prevention of ischaemic heart disease in men at increased risk. The Medical Research Council's General Practice Research Framework. Lancet 1998;351:233–241.

29 Hansson L, Zanchetti A, Carruthers SG, et al: Effects of intensive blood-pressure lowering and low-dose aspirin in patients with hypertension: principal results of the Hypertension Optimal Treatment (HOT) randomised trial. HOT Study Group. Lancet 1998;351:1755–1762.

30 CAPRIE Steering Committee: A randomized, blinded, trial of clopidogrel versus aspirin in patients at risk of ischaemic events (CAPRIE). Lancet 1996; 348:1329–1339.

31 Diener HC, Cunha L, Forbes C, Sivenius J, Smets P, Lowenthal A: European Stroke Prevention Study. 2. Dipyridamole and acetylsalicylic acid in the secondary prevention of stroke. J Neurol Sci 1996;143:1–13.

32 Kennedy J, Hill MD, Ryckborst KJ, Eliasziw M, Demchuk AM, Buchan AM; FASTER Investigators: Fast assessment of stroke and transient ischemic attack to prevent early recurrence (FASTER): a randomised controlled pilot trial. Lancet Neurol 2007;6:961–969.

33 Sacco RL, Diener H-C, Yusuf S, et al: Aspirin and extended-release dipyridamole versus clopidogrel for recurrent stroke. N Engl J Med 2008;359:1238–1251.

34 Wang Y, Zhao X, Liu L, et al: Clopidogrel with aspirin in acute minor stroke or transient ischemic attack. N Engl J Med 2013;369:11–19.

Pistoia · Sacco · Ornello · Degan · Tiseo · Carolei

35 Diener HC, Bogousslavsky J, Brass LM, et al: Aspirin and clopidogrel compared with clopidogrel alone after ischemic stroke or transient ischaemic attack in high-risk patients (MATCH): randomized, double-blind, placebo-controlled trial. Lancet 2004;364:331–337.

36 Bhatt DL, Fox KA, Hacke W, et al: Clopidogrel and aspirin versus aspirin alone for the prevention of atherothrombotic events. N Engl J Med 2006;354:1706–1717.

37 The ESPRIT Study Group, Halkes PH, van Gijn J, Kappelle LJ, Koudstaal PJ, Algra A: Aspirin plus dipyridamole versus aspirin alone after cerebral ischaemia of arterial origin (ESPRIT): randomised controlled trial. Lancet 2006;367:1665–1673.

38 Mant J, Hobbs FD, Fletcher K, et al: Warfarin versus aspirin for stroke prevention in an elderly community population with atrial fibrillation (the Birmingham Atrial Fibrillation Treatment of the Aged Study, BAFTA): a randomised controlled trial. Lancet 2007;370:493–503.

39 Connolly SJ, Ezekowitz MD, Yusuf S, et al: Dabigatran versus warfarin in patients with atrial fibrillation. N Engl J Med 2009;361:1139–1151.

40 Patel MR, Mahaffey KW, Garg J, et al: Rivaroxaban versus warfarin in nonvalvular atrial fibrillation. N Engl J Med 2011;365:883–891.

41 Connolly SJ, Eikelboom J, Joyner C, et al: Apixaban in patients with atrial fibrillation. N Engl J Med 2011;364:806–817.

42 Granger CB, Alexander JH, McMurray JJ, et al: Apixaban versus warfarin in patients with atrial fibrillation. N Engl J Med 2011;365:981–992.

43 Giugliano RP, Ruff CT, Braunwald E, et al. Edoxaban versus warfarin in patients with atrial fibrillation. N Engl J Med 2013;369:2093–2104.

44 EAFT (European Atrial Fibrillation Trial) Study Group: Secondary prevention in non-rheumatic atrial fibrillation after transient ischaemic attack or minor stroke. Lancet 1993;342:1255–1262.

45 Berge E, Abdelnoor M, Nakstad PH, Sandset PM: Low molecular-weight heparin versus aspirin in patients with acute ischaemic stroke and atrial fibrillation: a double-blind randomised study. HAEST Study Group. Heparin in Acute Embolic Stroke Trial. Lancet 2000;355:1205–1210.

46 Executive Committee for the Asymptomatic Carotid Atherosclerosis Study: Endarterectomy for asymptomatic carotid artery stenosis. JAMA 1995;273:1421–1428.

47 MRC Asymptomatic Carotid Surgery Trial (ACST) Collaborative Group: Prevention of disabling and fatal strokes by successful carotid endarterectomy in patients without recent neurological symptoms: randomised controlled trial. Lancet 2004;363:1491–1502.

48 Hobson RW, Weiss DG, Fields WS, et al: Efficacy of carotid endarterectomy for asymptomatic carotid stenosis. The Veterans Affairs Cooperative Study Group. N Engl J Med 1993;328:221–227.

49 Yadav JS, Wholey MH, Kuntz RE, et al; Stenting and Angioplasty with Protection in Patients at High Risk for Endarterectomy Investigators: Protected carotid-artery stenting versus endarterectomy in high-risk patients. N Engl J Med 2004;351:1493–1501.

50 Brott TG, Hobson RW 2nd, Howard G, et al: Stenting versus endarterectomy for treatment of carotid-artery stenosis. N Engl J Med 2010;363:11–23.

51 European Carotid Surgery Trialists' Collaborative Group (ECST): MRC European Carotid Surgery Trial: interim results for symptomatic patients with severe (70–99%) or with mild (0–29%) carotid stenosis. Lancet 1991;337:1235–1243.

52 North American Symptomatic Carotid Endarterectomy Trial. Methods, patient characteristics, and progress. Stroke 1991;22:711–720.

53 Mayberg MR, Wilson SE, Yatsu F, et al: Carotid endarterectomy and prevention of cerebral ischemia in symptomatic carotid stenosis. Veterans Affairs Cooperative Studies Program 309 Trialist Group. JAMA 1991;266:3289–3294.

54 Hoffmann A, Engelter S, Taschner C, et al: Carotid artery stenting versus carotid endarterectomy – a prospective randomised controlled single-centre trial with long-term follow up (BACASS). Schweiz Arch Neurol Psychiatr 2008;159:84–89.

55 Mas JL, Chatellier G, Beyssen B, et al: Endarterectomy versus stenting in patients with symptomatic severe carotid stenosis. N Engl J Med 2006;355:1660–1671.

56 Bonati LH, Jongen LM, Haller S, Flach HZ, Dobson J, Nederkoorn PJ; ICSS MRI Study Group: New ischemic brain lesions on MRI after stenting or endarterectomy for symptomatic carotid stenosis: a substudy of the International Carotid Stenting Study (ICSS). Lancet Neurol 2010;9:353–362.

57 SPACE Collaborative Group: 30 day results from the SPACE trial of stent-protected angioplasty versus carotid endarterectomy in symptomatic patients: a randomised non-inferiority trial. Lancet 2006;368:1239–1247.

58 Chimowitz MI, Lynn MJ, Howlett-Smith H, et al: Comparison of warfarin and aspirin for symptomatic intracranial arterial stenosis. N Engl J Med 2005;352:1305–1316.

59 Chimowitz MI, Lynn MJ, Derdeyn CP, et al: Stenting versus aggressive medical therapy for intracranial arterial stenosis. N Engl J Med 2011;365:993–1003.

60 International Classification of Functioning Disability and Health: ICF. Geneva, World Health Organization, 2001.

61 Lees KR, Bath PM, Schellinger PD, et al: Contemporary outcome measures in acute stroke research: choice of primary outcome measure. Stroke 2012;43:1163–1170.

62 Quinn TJ, Dawson J, Walters MR, Lees KR: Functional outcome measures in contemporary stroke trials. Int J Stroke 2009;4:200–205.

63 Asplund K: Clinimetrics in stroke research. Stroke 1987;18:528–530.

64 McDowell I, Newell C: Measuring Health: A Guide to Rating Scales and Questionnaires, ed 2. New York, Oxford University Press, 1996.

65 Banks JL, Marotta CA: Outcomes validity and reliability of the modified Rankin scale: implications for stroke clinical trials: a literature review and synthesis. Stroke 2007;38:1091–1096.

66 Brott T, Adams HP Jr, et al: Measurements of acute cerebral infarction: a clinical examination scale. Stroke 1989;20:864–870.

67 Goldstein LB, Bertels C, Davis J: Interrater reliability of the NIH stroke scale. Arch Neurol 1989;46:660–662.

68 Meyer BC, Hemmen TM, Jackson CM, Lyden PD: Modified National Institutes of Health Stroke Scale for use in stroke clinical trials: prospective reliability and validity. Stroke 2002;33:1261–1266.

69 Quinn TJ, Langhorne P, Stott DJ: Barthel Index for stroke trials: development, properties, and application. Stroke 2011; 42:1146–1151.

70 Lai SM, Duncan PW: Stroke recovery profile and the modified Rankin assessment. Neuroepidemiology 2001;20:26–30.

71 Appelros P, Terént A: Characteristics of the National Institute of Health Stroke Scale: results from a population-based stroke cohort at baseline and after one year. Cerebrovasc Dis 2004;17:21–27.

72 Kasner SE: Clinical interpretation and use of stroke scales. Lancet Neurol 2006; 5:603–612.

73 Ali M, Bath PM, Curram J, et al: The Virtual International Stroke Trials Archive. Stroke 2007;38:1905–1910.

74 Saver JL, Johnston KC, Homer D, et al: Infarct volume as a surrogate or auxiliary outcome measure in ischemic stroke clinical trials. The RANTTAS Investigators. Stroke 1999;30:293–298.

75 Engelter ST, Provenzale J, Petrella JR, DeLong DM, Alberts MJ: Infarct volume on apparent diffusion coefficient maps correlates with length of stay and outcome after middle cerebral artery stroke. Cerebrovasc Dis 2003;15:188–191.

76 Rosso C, Samson Y: The ischemic penumbra: the location rather than the volume of recovery determines outcome. Curr Opin Neurol 2014;27:35–41.

77 Ostergaard L, Jónsdóttir KY, Mouridsen K: Predicting tissue outcome in stroke: new approaches. Curr Opin Neurol 2009;22:54–59.

78 Schulz KF, Altman DG, Moher D; CONSORT Group: CONSORT 2010 Statement: updated guidelines for reporting parallel group randomised trials. J Clin Epidemiol 2010;63:834–840.

79 Dwan K, Gamble C, Williamson PR, Kirkham JJ; Reporting Bias Group: Systematic review of the empirical evidence of study publication bias and outcome reporting bias – an updated review. PLoS One 2013;8:e66844.

80 Tilley BC, Marler J, Geller NL, et al: Use of a global test for multiple outcomes in stroke trials with application to the National Institute of Neurological Disorders and Stroke t-PA Stroke Trial. Stroke 1996;27:2136–2142.

Francesca Pistoia, MD, PhD
Assistant Professor of Neurorehabilitation, Neurological Institute
Department of Biotechnological and Applied Clinical Sciences, University of L'Aquila
Via Vetoio, Coppito II
IT–67100 L'Aquila (Italy)
E-Mail francesca.pistoia@univaq.it

Beghi E, Logroscino G (eds): The Right Therapy for Neurological Disorders. From Randomized Trials to Clinical Practice.
Front Neurol Neurosci. Basel, Karger, 2016, vol 39, pp 71–80 (DOI: 10.1159/000445414)

Age, Comorbidity, Frailty in Observational and Analytic Studies of Neurological Diseases

Jan Novy[a] · Josemir W. Sander[b–d]

[a]Department of Clinical Neurosciences, Centre Hospitalier Universitaire Vaudois (CHUV) and University of Lausanne, Lausanne,
Switzerland; [b]NIHR University College London Hospitals Biomedical Research Centre, Department of Clinical and Experimental
Epilepsy, UCL Institute of Neurology, London, and [c]Epilepsy Society, Chalfont St. Peter, UK; [d]Stichting Epilepsie Instellingen
Nederland (SEIN), Heemstede, The Netherlands

Abstract

Background: Comorbidities are rarely taken into account
in studies of neurological conditions although they may
be a confounder of the outcome and treatment. The relationship between comorbidities and neurological conditions is also problematic as comorbidities may be
symptoms of the underlying cause of the neurologic condition or long-term adverse effects of the treatment.
Summary: There is evidence that several common neurological conditions have an increased burden of somatic and psychiatric comorbidities compared with matched
samples from the general population. Depression is
probably the most common comorbidity. Both psychiatric and somatic comorbidities have been shown to account for some of the premature mortality encountered
in these neurological conditions. Comorbidities and age
can also be important factors in the response and toler-
ance to treatment, and can alter the general outcome of
a disease. ***Key Messages:*** Age and comorbidities should
not be overlooked in the observation and assessment of
neurological conditions and their treatment.

© 2016 S. Karger AG, Basel

The importance of age and comorbidity has long
been recognized as influencing the overall outcome in medical conditions, but little attention
has been paid to this aspect in neurological conditions in treatment trials. According to Feinstein's
[1] original definition, 'the term comorbidity will
refer to any distinct additional clinical entity that
has existed or that may occur during the clinical
course of a patient who has the index disease under study'. Ageing and comorbidity often go together (but not invariably) as the proportion of
chronic conditions and multimorbidities in the
general population increases with ageing [2],
and this frequently coincides with an increased
mortality rate. The comorbidity effect is difficult to consider as a whole because of the heterogeneity of the conditions it encompasses and their
interindividual varying severity. The consequences of the overall burden of comorbidities have
mostly been studied in the mortality risk field;
several scores (such as the Charlson or Elixhauser
scores) were developed based on longitudinal

observational studies to predict the mortality risk over a period of time for combinations of comorbidities. Each comorbidity is given a weighted score according to the mortality risk observed associated with that comorbidity.

Treatment trials in neurological conditions rarely take comorbidities into account. Treatment trials favor homogenous cohorts, with well-defined age groups and disease severity, and tend to exclude people with problematic comorbidities, to give the greatest likelihood of showing a difference in outcome between comparators. Comorbidities could be confounders in several aspects of treatment trials [1]. As seen most obviously in studies where the outcome is survival, serious unrecognized comorbid conditions (e.g. cardiovascular diseases) can interfere with the results of the treatment trial. If comorbidities lead the individual to consult a physician, it is possible that the first signs of the studied disease, still unnoticed by the individual, could be identified and the diagnosis of the disease made earlier than usual in the natural history. If the comorbid condition's prognosis is poor, this may also bias the choice of treatment of the condition studied. Alternatively, even if a comorbid condition is not considered as relevant to the vital prognosis, it may contraindicate a specific therapy. Intellectual disabilities and significant psychiatric comorbidities may also prevent the full assessment of the outcome of the trial if there are no objective measurable results available as outcomes. Some of these issues can be addressed by randomization; those studies are, however, likely to exclude several important groups of patients, such as elderly people, those with multiple comorbidities, and people with intellectual disabilities or with psychiatric conditions.

Several causes of bias may also exist between comorbid conditions and the disease being considered. Comorbidities may result from long-term exposure to the medication of the studied disease. In some conditions, such as epilepsy, that are actually the symptom of an underlying cause, the underlying cause may at times be considered a comorbidity (e.g. brain tumor in epilepsy), or the comorbidity may be another manifestation (with the studied disease) of the underlying process. Some comorbidities (e.g. stroke) may also be risk factors of the studied disease. Comorbid conditions may also arise from the consequence of neurological conditions (e.g. traumatic lesions due to falls).

We will review comorbidities of some major neurological conditions and how they can influence the treatment and outcome of the principal neurological conditions.

Association between Neurological Conditions and Comorbidities

In the general population, adults were reported to have a median of two chronic health conditions with up to six in people older than 65 years [1]; these figures vary greatly according the methodology used and population studied [3, 4]. Consequently co-occurrence of several medical conditions is expected to be found not uncommonly in the general population and might raise the question of coincidental findings when studying comorbidities of a given condition. The association with comorbid conditions could also potentially be biased by the comparison of people seeing a physician regularly with people without medical follow-up. Some authors [5] have compared this phenomenon to Berkson's bias. This bias [6] suggests that people with two conditions are overrepresented in clinical care settings (in terms of hospitalization or outpatient clinic time) than would be expected from the combination of both conditions considered individually. Similarly, people followed by physicians for a medical condition could be more likely to receive and report the diagnosis of other disorders because of their greater contact with medical care services. This form of bias is also referred to as 'medical diagnosis bias' [5]. Hypothesizing that the increased burden of somatic comorbidities is fully related to reporting bias, health care utilization/costs as well as the premature mortality due to comorbidities in people with neurological conditions would not be expected to be significantly different from the general population. This is, however, clearly not the case, as health care utilization for comorbid conditions was shown to be increased in several neurological conditions such as epilepsy [7] or Parkinson's disease [8], or to contribute to a significant part of the total health care utilization in multiple sclerosis [9]. Premature mortality was demonstrated to be also directly linked with comorbidities in epilepsy (excluding its underlying cause) [10, 11], and there are similar suggestions for multiple sclerosis [12] and Parkinson's disease [13].

These data suggest that the association between neurological conditions and comorbid conditions is not limited to coincidental findings or reporting biases, but represent a genuine biological association [14].

Comorbidities in Neurological Conditions

Psychiatric conditions, especially depression, are probably the most common comorbidities associated with neurological conditions. Psychiatric comorbidities are common in people with multiple sclerosis [15]. People with multiple sclerosis, for instance, have a lifetime incidence of depression up to 50%, which is almost threefold more than the incidence of depression in the general population. If only the previous 12 months are taken into account, the prevalence of depression is twice that of the reported prevalence in the general population [2]. The lifetime incidence of anxiety disorders in people with multiple sclerosis is also similarly increased with incidence as high as 35% in people with multiple sclerosis. Depression is also common in all stages of stroke recovery and seems not to be related to the location of the stroke [16].

Several population-based studies [17–19] have shown that people with epilepsy have a higher prevalence of depression than the general population: 20–40% of people with epilepsy have major depression [20]. The prevalence of depression in people with refractory epilepsy in referral centers is probably higher than in people with epilepsy in the community. Treatment with antiepileptic drugs is a major confounder (as some medication may worsen mood disorders), but longitudinal follow-up studies have shown that the incidence of suicide attempts is highest shortly before the initiation of antiepileptic medication and decreases thereafter. This suggests that depression is linked with epilepsy rather than its treatment.

The prevalence of depression was also shown to be increased in people with migraine compared with the general population or people with other medical conditions [21]; even after correcting for age, gender and other chronic health conditions, people with migraine showed a 1.6 times increased risk of developing a major depressive episode compared with the general population [22]. Depression is also a major comorbidity of Parkinson's disease; it is widely accepted that almost every second person with Parkinson's disease will develop depression during the course of their disease [23]. The symptoms may be episodic or may persist in the longer term; milder episodes are very common. Cross-sectional studies in people with Parkinson's disease have shown that a quarter of them have a major depressive episode. Depression in Parkinson's disease does not seem to be explained by reactional factors as it does not parallel the motor course of the disease.

Further to this increased prevalence of depression in neurological disease, there is an intimate relationship between several diseases and depression. Several conditions such as epilepsy and migraine show a bidirectional association with depression [24, 25]; longitudinal studies have shown that having depression increases the incidence rate of those neurological conditions and conversely that having those neurological diseases increases the rate of depression. This bidirectional association suggests common risk factors underlying both depression and those neurological conditions. In other conditions such as in Parkinson's disease, depression has been suggested to be related to discrete loss of noradrenergic and serotonergic neurons as well as degeneration of dopaminergic neurons [23], while other authors have suggested that it may be the neurobiological counterpart of impulse control disorders [26].

Comorbidities in neurological conditions are not limited to psychiatric conditions; several neurological conditions have been shown to be associated with somatic comorbidities. Several community studies using either self-reported diagnoses or registers have shown a higher prevalence and incidence of somatic conditions in people with epilepsy than in the general population (table 1) [19]. This increase is not limited to specific somatic comorbidities, but affects the majority of conditions assessed in each study (table 1). This increased prevalence of somatic comorbidities is not fully explained by unfavorable socioeconomic factors among people with epilepsy. People with epilepsy have greater utilization of health care services for comorbid conditions [27], and necessitate higher health care costs than the general population after excluding epilepsy-related costs [28]. Migraine with aura, for instance, was shown to have a bidirectional association with epilepsy [29, 30], suggesting common underlying risk factors with epilepsy.

Migraine [31] has also been shown to be associated with several somatic comorbidities. A number of studies have suggested an increase in prevalence and incidence of stroke in both women and men [32]. Similarly, other cardiovascular conditions, such as ischemic heart disease (with an up to threefold increase) have been shown to be increased in people with migraine [33]. The prevalence of restless legs syndrome was found to be significantly higher in people with migraine than in people with tension or cluster headache [34]. Two studies have suggested that people with migraine are at a higher risk of obesity [35]. Several studies have suggested an association with irritable bowel syndrome. People with migraine were also found to have twice as many sleep problems as relatives without migraine, independent of potential psychiatric symptoms [36]. Somnambulism has also been suggested as being specifically associated with migraine rather than with other types of headache. One study [37] suggested that pregnant women with migraine would be at higher risk of adverse pregnancy outcomes than matched controls, with an increase approaching threefold. People with migraine, however, do not seem to have an increased prevalence of cancer, in particular women with migraine and gynecological cancer.

There have been some suggestions that people with multiple sclerosis also have an increased burden of concurrent somatic conditions [15]. A Dutch study using a national register [38] found an increased prevalence of liver and gallbladder disorders and of other unclassified conditions among the 31 comorbidities assessed among people with multiple sclerosis when compared with the general population. Liver test disturbances can, however, be due to interferon treatment. The prevalence of diabetes was significantly lower than in the general population. One systematic study [39], using a register validated with medical records review, found that people with multiple sclerosis were significantly more likely to have inflammatory bowel disease, irritable bowel syndrome, or migraine. Another study using self-reported diagnoses found a high frequency of hypercholesterolemia (37%), hypertension (30%), arthritis (16%), irritable bowel syndrome (13%), and chronic lung disease (13%), after correction for demographic factors; many comorbidities seemed, however, to occur at a similar frequency to the general population [15]. Findings about the prevalence of autoimmune diseases are conflicting – possibly because of differences in study design [15]. In two population-based studies, people with inflammatory bowel disease had an increased risk of incidence and prevalence of demyelinating disease, suggesting an association. In several small studies, co-occurrence of rheumatoid arthritis and multiple sclerosis was higher than expected. Some studies have also suggested that systemic lupus erythematosus occurs more frequently in people with multiple sclerosis than that expected in the general population. Thyroid disease was also reported as being not uncommon in people with multiple sclerosis, though the results of the different studies were conflicting. One recent study suggested that people with multiple sclerosis have an increased incidence of circulatory conditions, especially within the first years after diagnosis [40]. Epilepsy was also found significantly more frequently in people with multiple sclerosis, which is in line with the potential etiological role of multiple sclerosis in epilepsy.

Some studies have found an increased overall prevalence of comorbid conditions in Parkinson's disease, but statistical significance was not reached in many of the conditions assessed [41]. It has been suggested that some conditions frequently encountered in people with Parkinson's disease, such as REM sleep behavior disorder or dementia, share the same pathophysiologic mechanisms. There is some controversy about the risk of occurrence of cancer in Parkinson's disease with some studies showing a clear increase and others finding the opposite. There is also conflicting evidence on the potential association of diabetes and Parkinson's disease, while a majority of studies also show no increase or a relatively lower prevalence of hypertension in people with Parkinson's disease. There is conflicting evidence on the prevalence of cerebrovascular and ischemic heart disease. One study suggested that people with Parkinson's disease have a significantly higher prevalence of polyneuropathy, with the neuropathy related to B_{12} vitamin deficiency. There was a correlation between B_{12}

Table 1. Increased burden of comorbidities in people with epilepsy in the community (reproduced with permission [19])

All individuals	Rate ratio (95% CI)
Mental health disorders	
Neuroses	1.90 (1.79–2.02)
Obsessive-compulsive disorder	2.57 (1.61–4.10)
Anxiety	1.99 (1.85–2.14)
Hysteria	3.92 (2.55–6.04)
Depression	1.98 (1.87–2.09)
Schizophrenia	4.13 (3 .05–5.61)
Organic psychoses	6.05 (5.13–7.14)
Other psychoses	3.98 (3.62–4.38)
Alcohol dependence	5.70 (4.84–6.71)
Dementia	6.34 (5.47–7.35)
Somatic disorders	
CVA	6.96 (6.38–7.60)
Hemorrhagic CVA	10.62 (6.52–17.32)
Occlusive CVA	7.49 (5.69–9.86)
Transient ischemic attack	4.94 (4.44–5.50)
Neoplasia	1.05 (0.89–1.25)
Brain neoplasms	55.05 (38.00–79.75)
Meningiomas	31.44 (9.16–107.91)
Cerebral degeneration	6.80 (5.96–7.76)
Alzheimer's disease	8.05 (5.89–11.00)
Parkinson's disease	3.19 (2.44–4.18)
Migraine	1.60 (1.43–1.80)
Ischemic heart disease	1.34 (1.19–1.50)
Heart failure	1.68 (1.45–1.95)
Congenital cardiac abnormalities	7.34 (4.58–11.75)
Diabetes mellitus	1.57 (1.39–1.78)
Pneumonias	3.19 (2.72–3.74)
Asthma	1.30 (1.19–1.41)
Chronic bronchitis	1.67 (1.26–2.21)
Emphysema	1.25 (0.67–2.34)
Peptic ulcers	1.92 (1.55–2.37)
GI bleed	3.37 (2.78–4.08)
Upper GI bleed	4.31 (3.41–5.46)
Lower GI bleed	2.16 (1.43–3.25)
Unspecified GI bleed	2.85 (1.77–4.59)
Rheumatoid arthritis	0.99 (0.67–1.47)
Osteoarthritis	1.02 (0.91–1.15)
Fractures	2.17 (2.00–2.35)
Eczema	0.90 (0.47–1.74)

Prevalence of each condition was assessed in a general practitioners' register with a total cohort of 1,041,643 people. Though some conditions like brain tumor or stroke are likely to be biased by a causal association with epilepsy, most conditions assessed here were found to be increased in people with epilepsy. CVA = Cerebrovascular accident; GI = gastrointestinal.

vitamin deficiency and levodopa cumulative exposure, suggesting that the neuropathy might be treatment induced [42].

Effect of Comorbidities on Outcome and Treatment of Neurological Conditions

There are no systematic studies on the effect of comorbidities on neurological conditions, but there are suggestions that comorbid conditions can influence the outcome of several neurological conditions. Comorbidities may also influence the treatment and response to therapy.

Comorbidities were shown to have an impact on the mortality rate of people with neurological conditions. As well as having a greater prevalence of depression than the general population, people with epilepsy were shown to be at a higher suicide risk [43]. In Parkinson's disease, despite a high cumulative prevalence of depression, the suicide risk does not seem to be markedly increased, although people treated with deep brain stimulation may be at particular risk [44]. People who had a stroke are also at increased risk of suicide, which does not seem to be directly related to the severity of the episode, although disabilities in severe stroke may prevent the possibility of committing suicide [45]. The suicide rate is also significantly increased in people with multiple sclerosis, especially in the first years after the diagnosis, though again disabilities may prevent suicide later in the course of the disease.

The burden of somatic comorbidities also leads to premature mortality in several neurological conditions. People with epilepsy have an increased mortality rate even after excluding sudden unexpected death in epilepsy, which is linked with seizures. People with epilepsy have a two- to threefold increased mortality rate even up to 20 years after the diagnosis was established [10]. There are, however, several confounders such as the underlying cause of epilepsy and the potential long-term effects of its treatment. Despite these biases, there is evidence that people with epilepsy are more likely to die prematurely due to cerebrovascular disease – even people without a stroke before epilepsy onset [46] and regardless of treatment exposure [47]. People with epilepsy are at risk of premature mortality due to cancers other than brain tumors, and due to cardio- and cerebrovascular disease [10].

The role of comorbidities in Parkinson's disease mortality is also unclear. Some studies have suggested that the role of comorbidities (diabetes, hypertension, chronic obstructive pulmonary disease, osteoarthritis, stroke, and heart disease) is negligible. Others [48] have found significantly increased mortality rates due to cerebrovascular disease, respiratory disease, and ischemic heart disease. It was not clear, however, whether vascular parkinsonism could have been diagnosed as idiopathic Parkinson's disease in this community study. People with multiple sclerosis also have high mortality rates from comorbid conditions such as cardiovascular diseases [49].

In clinical practice, the choice of a particular treatment is often guided by the general medical needs (thus comorbidities) of the person. If a particular treatment, along with its main effect, has properties that may be beneficial to a comorbid condition, it may be preferred to a usual standard treatment option of the main disease. For instance, if a treatment has antidepressive properties, it may be preferred in a person with major depression. Conversely, a treatment may not be chosen if it has properties that may worsen a comorbid condition.

There are also suggestions that comorbidities and age can influence treatment outcome in neurological diseases and interfere with the symptoms of the disease. Age is well known as influencing the treatment of Parkinson's disease in terms of cognitive side effects induced by dopaminergic agonists, similarly to the anticholinergic medication used for tremor-dominant forms. Conversely, younger age at Parkinson's disease onset, longer disease duration, and male gender have been shown to be risk factors for dopaminergic dysregulation syndrome and impulse control disorders. Substance addiction and 'impulsive sensation seeking' personality traits were also shown to be risk factors. Ageing, independent from comorbid degenerative disease, was suggested as increasing the chance of remission of people with chronic epilepsy, probably by increasing the response to antiepileptic medication [11]. Obstructive sleep apnea may worsen epilepsy, possibly due to factors such as sleep deprivation, interference in sleep consolidation, and episodes of desaturation [50]. Obstructive sleep apnea was shown to be comorbid with epilepsy in up 33% of people with drug-resistant epilepsy, but higher seizure frequency has also been suggested as not being associated with obstructive sleep apnea [50]. Trials with continuous positive airway pressure suggest that correcting obstructive sleep apnea can improve epilepsy. A study [51] compared the epilepsy outcome of people with epilepsy and migraine compared with matched people with epilepsy only and found that, in the long term, people who had comorbid migraine were significantly less frequently seizure-free and were more frequently taking antiepileptic drug polytherapy. Recently, depression was also suggested to be associated with poor outcome in temporal lobe epilepsy surgery [52].

In multiple sclerosis, the absolute frequency of most autoimmune diseases is too low to have a substantial effect at the population level. Thyroid disease is more important because of its higher frequency and potential contribution to fatigue, a common symptom in multiple sclerosis [15]. Comorbidities may also interfere with the choice of treatment. The presence of a concomitant autoimmune condition associated with multiple sclerosis may preclude the use of natalizumab, as the use of an immunosuppressant (e.g. azathioprine) significantly increases the risk of developing progressive multifocal leukoencephalopathy [53]. Preexistence of uveitis in people with multiple sclerosis was shown to increase significantly the

incidence rate of fingolimod-associated macular edema with up to 20% of people developing this complication; diabetes was also a risk factor [54]. There are also suggestions that fingolimod should be used carefully in people with cardiovascular risk factors.

In migraine, it was suggested that obesity is an aggravating factor as it was shown to be associated with chronic daily headache, whereas this was not the case in tension-type headache [55]; other studies have found a correlation between obesity and the frequency of headaches. Others have wondered whether it may be the consequence of disturbed eating behavior due to more severe migraine, as found in experiment models [56]. The association with patent foramen ovale remains more controversial as some studies did not find any differences in its prevalence, whereas others found its closure could be an effective treatment of migraine [57].

An increased burden of psychiatric and somatic comorbidities is a common problem in people with neurological disease. As well as the morbidity they induce, they increase the long-term mortality rate independent of the neurological condition with which they are associated. In some situations, comorbidities and/or age also interfere with the treatment either in terms of efficacy or adverse events. The presence of comorbidities should not be underestimated. Despite heterogeneity, comorbidities should actively be taken into account when choosing a treatment and assessing its response.

Comorbidities in Randomized Controlled Trials

Randomized controlled trials rarely take into account comorbid conditions – indeed people with associated comorbidities are often excluded from such trials. This point raises the question of the generalizability of such studies in primary care where polymorbidity is commonplace [58]. Regulatory clinical trial data are indeed difficult to extrapolate to clinical practice as these studies are limited by their short duration, rigid inclusion (homogenous phenotype) and exclusion criteria (like comorbidities), inability to analyze the effect of concomitant medications, and lack of dosing flexibility [59]. Comorbidities may, as we discussed above, interfere with the outcome of the study, potentially leading to decreased power or even introducing a bias. A large review of randomized controlled trials found that 81% of potential participants were excluded because of comorbid conditions [60]. The most common approach to infer the validity a randomized controlled trial is checking inclusion and exclusion criteria and evaluating whether there are compelling reasons why the relative effect found in the trial results should not be applied to a specific patient group [61]. This approach assumes, however, that relative treatment effects demonstrated in randomized controlled trials would be stable across different populations which might not be the case [62]. To address this issue, some authors have suggested a shift in the design of randomized controlled trials towards a better characterization/stratification of comorbidities, cluster randomization, and wider interventions encompassing freedom to adjust the intervention according to the comorbidities [63]. Although these approaches would significantly increase the sample size needed to perform the study, they would also ease the recruitment of a wider population.

Acknowledgement

The authors wish to thank Dr. Myriam Schluep and Dr. Christian Wider for their help in the preparation of this chapter, and Dr. Gail Bell for reviewing the manuscript.

References

1 Feinstein AR: The pre-therapeutic classification of co-morbidity in chronic disease. J Chronic Dis 1970;23:455–468.

2 van den Akker M, Buntinx F, Metsemakers JF, Roos S, Knottnerus JA: Multimorbidity in general practice: prevalence, incidence, and determinants of co-occurring chronic and recurrent diseases. J Clin Epidemiol 1998;51:367–375.

3 Schellevis FG, van der Velden J, van de Lisdonk E, van Eijk JT, van Weel C: Comorbidity of chronic diseases in general practice. J Clin Epidemiol 1993;46:469–473.

4 Westert GP, Satariano WA, Schellevis FG, van den Bos GA: Patterns of comorbidity and the use of health services in the Dutch population. Eur J Public Health 2001;11:365–372.

5 Ottman R, Lipton RB, Ettinger AB, et al: Comorbidities of epilepsy: results from the Epilepsy Comorbidities and Health (EPIC) survey. Epilepsia 2011;52:308–315.

6 Feinstein AR, Walter SD, Horwitz RI: An analysis of Berkson's bias in case-control studies. J Chronic Dis 1986;39:495–504.

7 Gaitatzis A, Purcell B, Carroll K, Sander JW, Majeed A: Differences in the use of health services among people with and without epilepsy in the United Kingdom: socio-economic and disease-specific determinants. Epilepsy Res 2002;50:233–241.

8 Louis ED, Henchcliffe C, Bateman BT, Schumacher C: Young-onset Parkinson's disease: hospital utilization and medical comorbidity in a nationwide survey. Neuroepidemiology 2007;29:39–43.

9 Marrie RA, Elliott L, Marriott J, et al: Dramatically changing rates and reasons for hospitalization in multiple sclerosis. Neurology 2014;83:929–937.

10 Neligan A, Bell GS, Johnson AL, Goodridge DM, Shorvon SD, Sander JW: The long-term risk of premature mortality in people with epilepsy. Brain 2011;34:388–395.

11 Novy J, Belluzzo M, Caboclo LO, et al: The lifelong course of chronic epilepsy: the Chalfont experience. Brain 2013;136:3189–3199.

12 Ragonese P, Aridon P, Salemi G, D'Amelio M, Savettieri G: Mortality in multiple sclerosis: a review. Eur J Neurol 2008;15:123–127.

13 Driver JA, Kurth T, Buring JE, Gaziano JM, Logroscino G: Parkinson disease and risk of mortality: a prospective co-morbidity-matched cohort study. Neurology 2008;70:1423–1430.

14 Keezer MR, Sisodiya SM, Sander JW: Comorbidities of epilepsy: current concepts and future perspectives. Lancet Neurol 2016;15:106–115.

15 Marrie RA, Horwitz RI: Emerging effects of comorbidities on multiple sclerosis. Lancet Neurol 2010;9:820–828.

16 Hackett ML, Yapa C, Parag V, Anderson CS: Frequency of depression after stroke: a systematic review of observational studies. Stroke 2005;36:1330–1340.

17 Ettinger A, Reed M, Cramer J: Depression and comorbidity in community-based patients with epilepsy or asthma. Neurology 2004;63:1008–1014.

18 Tellez-Zenteno JF, Patten SB, Jetté N, Williams J, Wiebe S: Psychiatric comorbidity in epilepsy: a population-based analysis. Epilepsia 2007;48:2336–2344.

19 Gaitatzis A, Carroll K, Majeed A, W Sander J: The epidemiology of the comorbidity of epilepsy in the general population. Epilepsia 2004;45:1613–1622.

20 Gaitatzis A, Trimble MR, Sander JW: The psychiatric comorbidity of epilepsy. Acta Neurol Scand 2004;110:207–220.

21 Molgat CV, Patten SB: Comorbidity of major depression and migraine – a Canadian population-based study. Can J Psychiatry 2005;50:832–837.

22 Modgill G, Jette N, Wang JL, Becker WJ, Patten SB: A population-based longitudinal community study of major depression and migraine. Headache 2012;52:422–432.

23 Marsh L: Depression and Parkinson's disease: current knowledge. Curr Neurol Neurosci Rep 2013;13:1–9.

24 Breslau N, Lipton RB, Stewart WF, Schultz LR, Welch KM: Comorbidity of migraine and depression: investigating potential etiology and prognosis. Neurology 2003;60:1308–1312.

25 Kanner AM: Depression and epilepsy: a bidirectional relation? Epilepsia 2011;52(suppl 1):21–27.

26 Vriend C, Pattij T, van der Werf YD, et al: Depression and impulse control disorders in Parkinson's disease: two sides of the same coin? Neurosci Biobehav Rev 2014;38:60–71.

27 Copeland L, Ettinger AB, Zeber JE, Gonzalez JM, Pugh MJ: Psychiatric and medical admissions observed among elderly patients with new-onset epilepsy. BMC Health Serv Res 2011;11:84.

28 Ivanova JI, Birnbaum HG, Kidolezi Y, Qiu Y, Mallett D, Caleo S: Economic burden of epilepsy among the privately insured in the US. Pharmacoeconomics 2010;28:675–685.

29 Ludvigsson P, Hesdorffer D, Olafsson E, Kjartansson O, Hauser WA: Migraine with aura is a risk factor for unprovoked seizures in children. Ann Neurol 2006;59:210–213.

30 Lipton RB, Ottman R, Ehrenberg BL, Hauser WA: Comorbidity of migraine and epilepsy. Neurology 1994;44:2105–2110.

31 Wang SJ, Chen PK, Fuh JL: Comorbidities of migraine. Front Neurol 2010;1:16.

32 Stang PE, Carson AP, Rose KM, et al: Headache, cerebrovascular symptoms, and stroke: the Atherosclerosis Risk in Communities Study. Neurology 2005;64:1573–1577.

33 Rose KM, Carson AP, Sanford CP, et al: Migraine and other headaches: associations with Rose angina and coronary heart disease. Neurology 2004;63:2233–2239.

34 Chen PK, Fuh JL, Chen SP, Wang SJ: Association between restless legs syndrome and migraine. J Neurol Neurosurg Psychiatry 2010;81:524–528.

35 Peterlin BL, Rosso AL, Rapoport AM, Scher AI: Obesity and migraine: the effect of age, gender and adipose tissue distribution. Headache 2010;50:52–62.

36 Vgontzas A, Cui L, Merikangas KR: Are sleep difficulties associated with migraine attributable to anxiety and depression? Headache 2008;48:1451–1459.

37 Marozio L, Facchinetti F, Allais G, et al: Headache and adverse pregnancy outcomes: a prospective study. Eur J Obstet Gynecol Reprod Biol 2012;161:140–143.

38 Nuyen J, Schellevis FG, Satariano WA, et al: Comorbidity was associated with neurologic and psychiatric diseases: a general practice-based controlled study. J Clin Epidemiol 2006;59:1274–1284.

39 Marrie RA, Yu BN, Leung S, et al: The utility of administrative data for surveillance of comorbidity in multiple sclerosis: a validation study. Neuroepidemiology 2013;40:85–92.

40 Christiansen CF: Risk of vascular disease in patients with multiple sclerosis: a review. Neurol Res 2012;34:746–753.

41 Leibson CL, Maraganore DM, Bower JH, Ransom JE, O'brien PC, Rocca WA: Comorbid conditions associated with Parkinson's disease: a population-based study. Mov Disord 2006;21:446–455.

42 Rajabally YA, Martey J: Neuropathy in Parkinson disease: prevalence and determinants. Neurology 2011;77:1947–1950.

43 Pugh MJ, Hesdorffer D, Wang CP, et al: Temporal trends in new exposure to antiepileptic drug monotherapy and suicide-related behavior. Neurology 2013;81:1900–1906.

44 Voon V, Krack P, Lang AE, et al: A multicentre study on suicide outcomes following subthalamic stimulation for Parkinson's disease. Brain 2008;131:2720–2728.

45 Teasdale TW, Engberg AW: Suicide after a stroke: a population study. J Epidemiol Community Health 2001;55:863–866.

46 Trinka E, Bauer G, Oberaigner W, Ndayisaba JP, Seppi K, Granbichler CA: Cause-specific mortality among patients with epilepsy: results from a 30-year cohort study. Epilepsia 2013;54:495–501.

47 Olesen JB, Abildstrøm SZ, Erdal J, et al: Effects of epilepsy and selected antiepileptic drugs on risk of myocardial infarction, stroke, and death in patients with or without previous stroke: a nationwide cohort study. Pharmacoepidemiol Drug Saf 2011;20:964–971.

48 Ben-Shlomo Y, Marmot MG: Survival and cause of death in a cohort of patients with parkinsonism: possible clues to aetiology? J Neurol Neurosurg Psychiatry 1995;58:293–299.

49 Brønnum-Hansen H, Koch-Henriksen N, Stenager E: Trends in survival and cause of death in Danish patients with multiple sclerosis. Brain 2004;127:844–850.

50 Foldvary-Schaefer N, Andrews ND, Pornsriniyom D, Moul DE, Sun Z, Bena J: Sleep apnea and epilepsy: who's at risk? Epilepsy Behav 2012;25:363–367.

51 Velioğlu SK, Boz C, Özmenoğlu M: The impact of migraine on epilepsy: a prospective prognosis study. Cephalalgia 2005;25:528–535.

52 Cleary RA, Thompson PJ, Fox Z, Foong J: Predictors of psychiatric and seizure outcome following temporal lobe epilepsy surgery. Epilepsia 2012;53:1705–1712.

53 Kappos L, Bates D, Hartung HP, et al: Natalizumab treatment for multiple sclerosis: recommendations for patient selection and monitoring. Lancet Neurol 2007;6:431–441.

54 Jain N, Bhatti MT: Fingolimod-associated macular edema: Incidence, detection, and management. Neurology 2012;78:672–680.

55 Bigal ME, Lipton RB: Obesity is a risk factor for transformed migraine but not chronic tension-type headache. Neurology 2006;67:252–257.

56 Ray ST, Kumar R: Migraine and obesity: cause or effect? Headache 2010;50:326–328.

57 Dowson A, Mullen MJ, Peatfield R, et al: Migraine Intervention with STARFlex Technology (MIST) trial: a prospective, multicenter, double-blind, sham-controlled trial to evaluate the effectiveness of patent foramen ovale closure with STARFlex septal repair implant to resolve refractory migraine headache. Circulation 2008;117:1397–1404.

58 Fortin M, Dionne J, Pinho G, Gignac J, Almirall J, Lapointe L: Randomized controlled trials: do they have external validity for patients with multiple comorbidities? Ann Fam Med 2006;4:104–108.

59 Sander JW: New antiepileptic drugs in practice – how do they perform in the real world? Acta Neurol Scand 2005;112: 26–29.

60 Van Spall HC, Toren A, Kiss A, Fowler RA: Eligibility criteria of randomized controlled trials published in high-impact general medical journals: a systematic sampling review. JAMA 2007;297: 1233–1240.

61 Post PN, de Beer H, Guyatt GH: How to generalize efficacy results of randomized trials: recommendations based on a systematic review of possible approaches. J Eval Clin Pract 2013;19:638–643.

62 Fuller J: Rationality and the generalization of randomized controlled trial evidence. J Eval Clin Pract 2013;19:644–647.

63 Smith SM, Bayliss EA, Mercer SW, et al: How to design and evaluate interventions to improve outcomes for patients with multimorbidity. J Comorbidity 2013;3:10–17.

Josemir W. Sander
NIHR University College London Hospitals Biomedical Research Centre
Department of Clinical and Experimental Epilepsy, UCL Institute of Neurology
Queen Square
London WC1N 3BG (UK)
E-Mail l.sander@ucl.ac.uk

Beghi E, Logroscino G (eds): The Right Therapy for Neurological Disorders. From Randomized Trials to Clinical Practice.
Front Neurol Neurosci. Basel, Karger, 2016, vol 39, pp 81–92 (DOI: 10.1159/000445417)

Disease Course, Outcome Measures, and Prognostic Predictors in Epilepsy: Opportunities for Improving Outcome of Drug Trials

Dieter Schmidt

Epilepsy Research Group, Berlin, Germany

Abstract

Background: A major concern over the development of new antiepileptic drugs (AEDs) is that the new AEDs have not added substantial clinical benefit over available antiseizure treatment. Additionally, current AEDs have neither improved the health of epilepsy patients nor been shown to prevent epilepsy or to improve the disease. **Summary:** This chapter reviews new data on patterns of epilepsy with remission and relapse, prognostic factors for seizure outcome, and innovative patient-related outcome measures. Applying this knowledge presents opportunities to improve the drug treatment of epilepsy. **Key Messages:** Patient-relevant outcome measures and trial designs may be optimized to provide both evidence for efficacy and safety of AEDs and, in addition, for added clinical benefit over existing treatment. Added benefit of a new AED may be shown by evidence of higher antiseizure efficacy, better health, shorter disease duration, fewer side effects, and improved quality of life compared to available standard treatment. Moving from largely patient-irrelevant outcome measures such as 50% seizure reduction or use of placebo controls to innovative comparison of new AEDs versus standard treatment will revitalize the clinical development of new antiseizure treatments. Hopefully this will usher in a new era of much-needed antiepileptogenic agents that prevent or improve the patterns of epilepsy.

Bringing a new antiepileptic drug (AED) from bench to bedside is a risky and expensive proposition [1]. The development of a new AED is estimated to cost many hundreds of millions of dollars; as a result, decisions about funding a drug development program are based as much on economics as on science and medicine [1]. Major pharmaceutical companies have lost interest in developing drugs for epilepsy and prefer to invest in other, seemingly more lucrative, treatment areas [1].

One important reason for the lower investment of industry in epilepsy is the difficulty and the high development costs to show substantial differences between the new compound and the available antiseizure treatment or, sometimes, even placebo [2]. Inconsistent treatment effects of the same compound during clinical development may require additional trials which will increase development costs. One reasonable explanation for poor efficacy outcome is that participants shared too many bad prognostic features or their epilepsy may have been on an unfavorable course at entry. Investment in the development of new compounds for epilepsy is not favored by the use of entrenched, largely patient-irrelevant outcome measures such as the 50% seizure reduction versus baseline, by the use of placebo controls, or by noninferiority trial design [2]. These outcomes cannot provide evidence for substantial added clinical benefit of the new AED [2]. Return on investment suffers because premium pricing is increasingly based on proving added clinical benefit over current treatment [1].

Given these serious challenges, it may be of interest to critically review recent insights into the disease course of epilepsy and prognostic predictors for seizure outcome, and to discuss clinically useful (and less useful) outcome measures in epilepsy. Finally, this chapter will critically examine whether enrichment of good prognostic features may be useful to improve outcome in epilepsy trials.

Patterns of Seizure Recurrence in the Course of Epilepsy

Longitudinal cohort studies of epilepsy with a follow-up over several decades have shown distinctive patterns of seizure outcome [3, 4]. In a study from Turku (Finland), 144 children were followed for a median of 37 years from the initiation of therapy (19–47 years; by enquiry every 5 years) [3]. The most striking result of the studies is that stationary patterns exist in approximately 70% of patients with new-onset epilepsy, including 50% who become seizure-free early and stay seizure-free until the end of follow-up. A further 20% will never be seizure-free for at least 1 year during long-term follow-up. The remaining 30% will either switch from being not seizure-free to seizure-free in 19% (late remission) or, unfortunately, in 14% from being seizure-free to becoming not seizure-free (late drug resistance) in the course of their epilepsy [3] (fig. 1).

Brodie et al. [5] have subsequently shown similar seizure patterns in their hospital-based cohort. Limitations of these long-term follow-up studies of a same-patient group going back 40 years or more include lack of treatment controls and lack of follow-up for those who preferred no treatment at entry. As a consequence, these studies cannot differentiate AED treatment effects from random fluctuations of seizures or the natural history of disease resulting in seizure remission and recurrence. Finally, new AEDs, MRI, CAT scans, and epilepsy surgery were not available at the time when the studies were started.

Are Antiepileptic Drugs Affecting Outcome Patterns in Epilepsy?

Only recently, an important pilot study in Dutch children tried to assess the effect of AED treatment on the patterns of uncontrolled epilepsy [6]. After diagnosis, 453 patients with childhood-onset epilepsy had a 5-year follow-up with regular visits and data collection. Intractability during the first 5 years was compared with that in the last year of follow-up. In this study, intractability was defined as having no 3-month remission during a 1-year period despite adequate medical treatment. The study identified 3 patient populations: those with only early intractability, those with only late intractability, and those with early and late intractability. According to the authors, AEDs were of little use in all three groups in preventing or stopping intractability whenever it occurred in the course of epilepsy [6]. The study

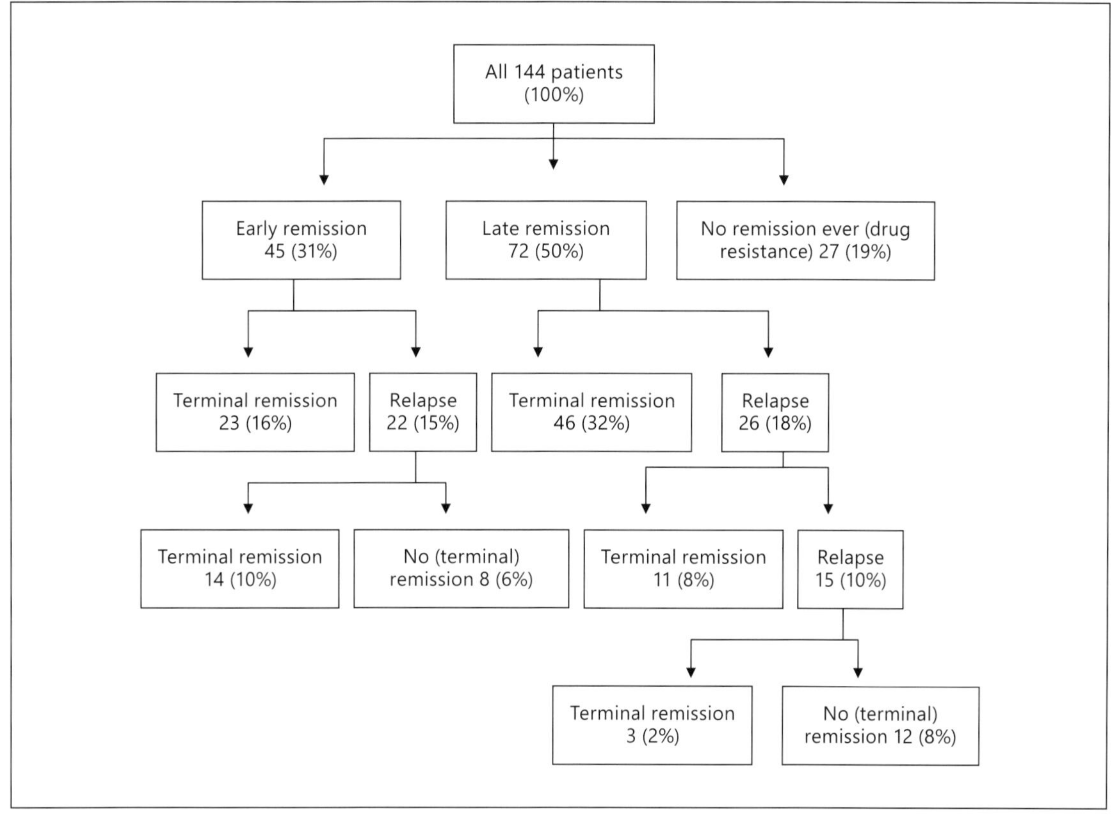

Fig. 1. Stable and intermittent patterns of seizure remission and relapse in the natural history of treated epilepsy. Most patients do follow a stable course by entering early remission and staying in remission until the end of follow-up (terminal remission, 48%), or less often by never entering remission (drug-resistant epilepsy 19%). In contrast, one third of newly treated patients with epilepsy have an intermittent pattern. Patients with an intermittent pattern may either enter late remission after experiencing seizures for many years (19%) or have seizures after years of entering early remission (14%). With permission from Sillanpää and Schmidt [3].

authors felt that the natural course of epilepsy probably best explained the observed patterns [6]. The study suggests that current AEDs do not seem to be able to improve the course of epilepsy; however, confirmation is needed.

Are Long-Term Epilepsy Patterns Affecting Seizure Outcome in Antiepileptic Drug Trials?

In controlled trials, efficacy and safety of new AEDs is usually assessed during a period of several months up to 1 year. Often the past history of the epilepsy is not well documented. Thus, it may be difficult to know at entry which patterns of epilepsy the participant actually is. It is easy to see that patients and physicians alike may wrongly attribute the disappearance of prior uncontrolled seizures to the assigned treatment, when, in reality, the trial outcome is actually reflecting a pattern of late remission. Likewise, late-onset uncontrolled seizures may be wrongly interpreted as failure of antiseizure medication when in fact it is the failure of current antiseizure treatment to prevent the pattern of late intractability. Of course, this is speculative and we

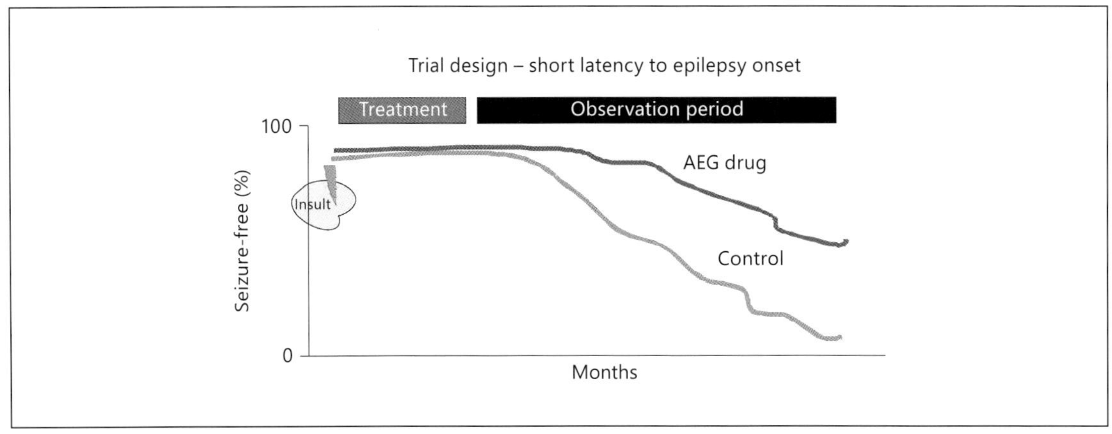

Fig. 2. Clinical testing of antiseizure effect, added clinical benefit, and an antiepileptogenic compound for epilepsy prevention in one trial. For an epileptogenic insult with rapid onset of epilepsy, participants could be randomized to receive AEG treatment or control (standard antiseizure treatment or placebo) for a period of time after the insult. Following withdrawal of the treatment, participants would be followed for the onset of seizures. If antiepileptogenic treatment is effective, the rate of developing unprovoked seizures would be lower in the AEG-treated group, providing evidence for an added clinical benefit in efficacy. For testing of a disease-modifying effect, patients with ongoing epilepsy can be randomized to a period of adjunctive treatment with an experimental antiepileptogenic agent with an adjunctive antiseizure agent as control. For assessment of added clinical benefit in quality of life or side-effect profile, extended testing during follow-up may be needed after withdrawal of the test agent and the control. With permission from Schmidt et al. [8].

need more data to confirm this concern. The problem is aggravated when a patient is participating in subsequent trials and the pattern changes over the years. Finally, it may be of great interest to identify predictors of the pattern of unrelenting drug-resistant epilepsy, which is seen in approximately 1 in 5 patients with new-onset epilepsy [3, 5] for assessing treatment for very severe epilepsy.

If a patient has an unstable pattern of remission and relapse, this may explain why one cannot reliably predict or expect better treatment outcome when re-exposing patients to an AED that had been successful in the past. Additionally, a fluctuating pattern of placebo response, if it exists, would stand in the way of the proposal to use historical controls to limit exposure to placebo in AED trials [7]. Studies are urgently needed to assess the variability of same-patient placebo response, if any, during long-term follow-up.

On a more positive note, the recognition of patterns of uncontrolled seizures and their remission might lead to a new class of drug treatment for epilepsy. Development of disease-modifying treatment may be able to prevent or improve seizure outcome in those with a pattern of late-onset drug-resistant epilepsy [1, 8, 9].

Finally, antiepileptogenic medication may one day be able to prevent the occurrence of epilepsy in those at risk and, hopefully, the onset of unrelenting drug-resistant epilepsy from the start [1, 8, 9]. The feasibility of testing a course of antiepileptogenic treatment hinges on the discovery of suitable agents and of biomarkers to predict which patient at risk will develop epilepsy and, ideally, the patterns of epilepsy [8]. This would open a new chapter on the drug treatment of epilepsy. We would move from currently purely symptomatic antiseizure relief to truly antiepileptogenic treatment that affects the underlying disease and its patterns (fig. 2).

When Is Epilepsy Cured?

Observational studies have shown that newly treated epilepsy has an often good prognosis with 65–85% of cases eventually entering long-term remission of 5 years or more, and an even higher proportion of cases entering a short-term remission [3–5]. For the many patients who are seizure-free for years on AEDs, often with their first AED, it is of great clinical interest whether epilepsy will remain in remission when AEDs are stopped and under which circumstances remission off AEDs represent cure of epilepsy.

Any attempt to determine cure is fraught with a number of problems. Ultimately, cure is proven when patients are in sustained remission off AEDs followed up to the end of their life. As this is not practical, cure of epilepsy is usually defined as sustained seizure remission continuing after discontinuation of AEDs [10]. The ILAE Task Force on the Definition of Epilepsy noted recently that no adequate data are available on seizure recurrence risk after being seizure-free and off medication for extended periods of time [11]. This assessment of the Task Force is a bit surprising as several studies have reported long-term remission off AED treatment in up to 81% depending on the population studied (see [10] for review). One example is a recent study that determined long-term seizure cure in a population-based cohort of 133 patients followed up since their first seizure before the age of 16 years [10]. Cure was defined in this study as remission off AEDs for a minimum of the last 5 years preceded by long-term remission on AEDs for many years. At the end of the 45-year follow-up (mean 39.8, median 44, range 11–47), 81 (61%) of 133 patients had entered at least 5-year remission off AEDs, thus meeting the definition of cure of this study. The 81 patients were seizure-free off AEDs for a mean of 34.4 years (median 38, range 6–46), and 59 (73%) of 81 following the first standard medication until the end of follow-up (mean 36.5, median 39, range 14–46 years) [10]. Furthermore,

the ILAE Task Force on the Definition of Epilepsy pointed out in their paper that delineation of circumstances in which epilepsy is definitively cured is beyond the scope of their paper [11].

Is 'Resolved Epilepsy' A Useful Concept?
The ILAE Task Force chose to define epilepsy as being resolved for individuals who had an age-dependent epilepsy syndrome but are now past the applicable age or those who have remained seizure-free for the last 10 years, with no seizure medicines for the last 5 years [11]. However, a critical commentary pointed out that the definition of 'resolved epilepsy' seems to be based on 'expert opinion' and seems arbitrary [12]. A person who is seizure-free for >10 years and off medications for 5 years still has an annual seizure recurrence risk of 0.5–1% [13–15]. This, it was argued, can be translated to a 10- to 20-fold increase in risk for an unprovoked seizure when compared to the general population [12]. It was suggested that the level of residual risk for further seizures would be a better starting point for a definition of resolved epilepsy (e.g. annual risk of 1%) [12]. This would allow for individualized determination of the time at which this definition is met, factoring in variables such as age, seizure type, and persistence or resolution of EEG abnormalities [12]. To address this valid concern, the concept of resolved epilepsy clearly needs further discussion and robust assessment.

Patient-Related Outcome Measures: Opportunity for Improvement?

The value of patient-centered outcome measures for improving the care and satisfaction of patients in several therapeutic areas is now well recognized, and patient-centered outcomes are increasingly being incorporated into clinical research. In epilepsy, however, trials in prior drug-resistant epilepsy continue to use largely patient-irrelevant outcome measures such as the 50% seizure reduction versus baseline and noninferiority outcome [2]. In addition, clinically irrelevant controls such as placebo are still used. Placebo is not validated for epilepsy treatment, yet placebo is still widely used and (justifiably) recognized by regulatory authorities [2]. A recent study showed that placebo response is highly heterogeneous between studies, even when analyzing trials of the same new AED [16]. A further serious concern is that placebo response is influenced by many clinical variables which are currently not well controlled in drug trials (see below).

In 1,106 adults and children with refractory epilepsy participating in placebo-controlled trials, the overall weighted pooled-risk difference in favor of AEDs over placebo for seizure freedom was only 6 and 21 for 50% seizure reduction [16]. These data show that the placebo-corrected efficacy of adjunctive treatment with modern AEDs is disappointingly small and suggests that better strategies of finding drugs are needed for refractory epilepsy, which is a major public health problem [16]. A clinically much more relevant way to assess the efficacy of new AEDs is to compare them to the efficacy of standard AEDs in a superiority design. In this way it will be possible to determine added clinical benefit of the new AED over available treatment, if it exists.

Assessing Added Clinical Benefits of Antiepileptic Drugs

Traditionally, the core strategy of the drug industry was to obtain a license based on superiority outcome for parameters of efficacy such as 50% seizure reduction or percent change of seizure frequency over baseline of adjunctive test drug versus placebo. This is considered justifiably as a legally and scientifically valid end point of efficacy in the US and the EU. If the requirements for efficacy and safety are met, the new compound is labeled as a legal therapeutic option. However, evidence that such therapy has added clinical benefit over standard treatment, which is of great interest to patients and physicians, currently is not part of the legal requirements for labelling of a new compound anywhere.

More recently, however, while accepting the traditional measure of efficacy to grant a license for marketing, several EU countries have passed legislation that pricing of the new compound depends on showing added clinical benefit of the test compound versus a well-chosen and agreed-on standard treatment (table 1). Essentially, added benefit is defined as better health, shorter disease duration, fewer side effects, and improved quality of life of the new AED over a standard treatment for the same indication as the new AED (table 1).

The choice of the standard treatment by the pharmaceutical company is crucial and may be contested by the authorities when assessing added clinical benefit. The new compound is only reimbursable at a higher price than the comparative standard AED when an added clinical benefit is shown after careful review of the dossier which the pharmaceutical company has submitted. Which outcome parameters are considered to show an added clinical benefit is negotiated between the pharmaceutical company and the authorities.

Prognostic Features: Opportunities for Improving Treatment Outcome?

Clinical factors associated with outcome in new-onset epilepsy have been well studied in longitudinal cohort studies of prognosis in epilepsy [e.g. 3, 4]. Factors consistently found to predict a worse outcome include the presence of a neurodeficit, high frequency of seizures before therapy, and some, mostly pediatric and uncommon, epilepsy syndromes [3, 4, 17] (table 2).

The likelihood of long-term remission of seizures is much better in newly diagnosed cases than in patients with chronic epilepsy [e.g. 3–5].

Table 1. Framework for assessing efficacy, safety, and added benefit of an AED

Assessment	Efficacy and safety (EMA, FDA)	Added benefit (IQWiG)
Preclinical trial design	Evidence of efficacy and safety vs. vehicle used for test drug in animal models of seizures	Differentiation in efficacy or safety of test AED vs. standard treatment in animal models of epilepsies or epilepsy syndromes
Clinical trial design (phase II and III)	Superiority of adjunctive test AED vs. with placebo control or intentionally less effective dose of AEDs (EMA, FDA); noninferiority design (EMA only); design to reduce the exposure to placebo (experimental stage)	Superiority of efficacy, safety design with standard treatment control for adjunctive treatment of prior refractory seizures and monotherapy in new-onset epilepsy; evidence for added benefit (definition see text); preferred use of patient-relevant outcome measures (see text)
Pricing	Pricing after determination of efficacy and safety (FDA)	Reimbursement and pricing is determined by the government following determination of added benefit

For definition of added benefit, see text. EMA = European Medicines Agency; FDA = US Food and Drug Administration; IQWiG = Institute for Quality and Efficiency in Healthcare (Germany).

The early response to treatment is a good guide to longer-term prognosis (although not inevitably so, as in a minority of cases seizure remission can develop after prolonged activity [e.g. 3, 4]). In addition to clinical features, pathological MRI results have been shown to be associated with a poor prognosis [18], while the role of EEG features for long-term prognosis is less clear [10].

A related question is whether a first remission of at least 5 years guarantees sustained remission. Although most patients with newly treated epilepsy who enter remission remain seizure-free, this is not inevitable. A recent study determined the likelihood of seizure relapse, remission following relapse, and premature retirement after entering the first seizure remission of 5 years or more in a population-based cohort of 115 medically treated patients [19]. The study patients were followed up from their first seizure during childhood for 42 years. Among 141 patients, 115 (82%) entered a first remission of at least 5 years. Although 69 (60%) of the 115 patients had no relapse, at least one seizure relapse was seen in 46 patients (40%) and 14 patients (12%) never re-entered 5-year remission. On multivariate

Table 2. Clinical factors predicting poor seizure outcome in multivariate analysis [modified from 17]

Disease-related factors
  Prior neonatal seizures
  Symptomatic etiology
  Abnormal intelligence
  Early childhood age at onset of epilepsy
  High pretreatment seizure frequency
  Tonic or simple partial seizures
  Complex partial or atonic seizures
  Diffuse slowing in EEG
  Focal spike and wave activity in EEG

Treatment-related factors
  High seizure frequency during early treatment
  Early response to therapy
  Number of seizures during 6 months following onset of epilepsy
  Delayed time to first remission seizure clustering during drug treatment

analysis of clinical features, cognitive impairment predicted seizure relapse for those entering their first remission of 5 years or more. Despite entering their first remission of 5 years or more, individuals with epilepsy face clinically important risks including relapse, failure to re-enter remission following relapse, and premature retirement. Cognitive impairment predicted seizure relapse [19].

Does Failure of the First Two Life-Time AEDs Predict a Poor Prognosis?
Given the grave morbidity and mortality of drug-resistant epilepsy, it is of great clinical interest to determine how often previously proven drug-resistant epilepsy is reversible without surgery and whether remission can be predicted by clinical features in children with incident drug-resistant epilepsy [20].

A recent study determined the likelihood of 1-, 2-, and 5-year seizure remission and terminal 5-year seizure remission after the first adequate drug regimen in a population-based cohort of 102 medically treated patients with incident epilepsy, i.e. first-ever occurrence of drug-resistant epilepsy, as defined by the International League against Epilepsy [21]. Among the 102 patients, 98 had focal seizures (68 symptomatic and 30 idiopathic/cryptogenic), 1 had generalized convulsive seizures, and 3 had unclassified seizures. At the end of the 40.5-year median follow-up from the onset of adequate medication before the age of 16 years, 84 patients (82%) with incident drug-resistant epilepsy eventually entered one or more 1-year remissions, 81 (79%) entered one or more 2-year remissions, 70 (69%) entered one or more 5-year remissions, and 52 (51%) entered 5-year terminal remissions. In contrast, 18 (18%) of the 102 patients with incident drug-resistant epilepsy never entered any 1-year remission, 21 (21%) never entered 2-year remission, 32 (31%) never entered 5-year remission, and 50 (49%) never entered any 5-year terminal remission [20].

On multivariate analysis of clinical features, in every remission category, idiopathic or cryptogenic etiology was the only significant predictor of entering remission. Incident drug-resistant epilepsy is eventually reversible in 49–79% of patients with mostly focal epilepsy, resulting in long-term remission of variable duration. Idiopathic or cryptogenic etiology is a clinical predictor of reversible drug-resistant epilepsy [20]. This study shows that a hypothetical trial that elected to include only those who meet the minimum requirement of drug-resistant epilepsy as defined by the ILAE in 2010 [21] can be expected to achieve 1-year remission in nearly 80% of cases. However, this does not guarantee a difference in efficacy of the test compound against a standard drug or placebo as a placebo response has not seemed to have been determined in such a population. A further limitation is that a positive trial would likely limit the labelling and the indication of the new AED to this restricted patient group and may make it difficult to generalize the finding. This may not favor investment in this trial design.

Do Patients with Seizure Clusters Have a Poorer Prognosis?
To provide evidence of whether seizure clustering is associated with drug resistance in childhood-onset epilepsy, a prospective, long-term population-based study was performed in 120 patients with an average follow-up of 37 years since their first seizure [22]. At the end of the follow-up period, 26 (11 boys) of these patients (22%) had recorded clusters of seizures. Fourteen recorded pretreatment clusters, including 10 patients with clusters as first seizures, and in 12 patients clusters occurred during treatment. In these 12 patients, the first clustering began after 16 (range 0–35; median 15) years of treatment. Compared with the patients without clusters, those with clusters more often had at least one seizure per week at the initial stage (63 vs. 32%, p = 0.0178) and during the follow-up period (p value varied from 0.0464 to 0.0064). Patients who had seizure clusters during drug therapy were more likely to have drug-resistant epilepsy compared to those not experiencing seizure clusters (42 vs. 13%; p = 0.0102) and had a lower rate of entering 5-year terminal remission (p = 0.0039) and 5-year remission (p = 0.0230). In contrast, patients with

seizure clustering prior to, but not during, treatment versus those with no clustering showed no difference in seizure outcome [22].

Does a Low Pretreatment Seizure Frequency Predict a Good Prognosis?

To address this question, factors predictive of long-term seizure and mortality outcome were determined in a population-based cohort of 144 patients followed up since their first seizure before the age of 16 years [23]. At the end of the 40-year follow-up, 117 (81%) of 144 patients had entered one or more 5-year remissions, including 23 patients who were seizure-free with the first adequate medication until the end of the follow-up. In contrast, 27 (19%) patients never experienced any 5-year remission (i.e. were drug-resistant by the definition used in this study). Two independent factors were found to be associated with long-term seizure outcome defined as entering 5-year remission: seizure frequency less than weekly versus weekly during 12 months preceding onset of AEDs [p = 0.0069, OR 21.5 (2.3–199.1)], and idiopathic/cryptogenic versus symptomatic etiology as determined by assessing neurological deficit or its absence [p = 0.0153, OR 6.3 (1.4–27.8)]. Patients with pretreatment seizure frequency of less than once a week and idiopathic or cryptogenic etiology had a threefold higher chance to remain seizure-free from the onset of the first adequate antiepileptic therapy until the end of follow-up compared with patients who had a high pretreatment seizure frequency and a symptomatic etiology (OR 3.4, 95% CI 1.2–9.2; p = 0.0162) [23].

Predictors of Cure

Clinical conditions of long-term cure in childhood-onset epilepsy, defined as sustained remission off AED treatment, are not well known. To address that clinically important question, a population-based study determined clinical factors predictive of long-term seizure cure in a population-based cohort of 133 patients followed up since their first seizure before the age of 16 years [10]. At the end of the 45-year follow-up (mean 39.8, median 44, range 11–47), 81 (61%) of 133 patients had entered at least 5-year remission among off AEDs, meeting the definition of cure of this study. The 81 patients were seizure-free off AEDs for a mean of 34.4 years (median 38, range 6–46), and 59 (73%) of 81 following the first standard medication until the end of follow-up (mean 36.5, median 39, range 14–46 years). Four independent factors were found to be associated with cure compared to having seizures on AEDs: seizure frequency less than weekly during the first 12 months of AED treatment (p = 0.002), pretreatment seizure frequency less than weekly (p = 0.002), higher IQ (>70; p = 0.021), and idiopathic or cryptogenic versus symptomatic etiology (p = 0.042). Patients with seizure frequency of less than once a week during early treatment and idiopathic etiology had a ninefold chance to enter cure since the onset of the first adequate antiepileptic therapy until the end of follow-up compared with patients who had at least weekly seizures on AEDs and a symptomatic etiology (RR 8.7, 95% CI 2.0–37.0; p < 0.001). In conclusion, IQ, etiology, and seizure frequencies both in the first year of AED treatment and prior to medication appear to be clinical predictors of cure in childhood-onset epilepsy [10].

Are Prognostic Features Available to Predict Placebo Response?

Because it is unethical to expose patients with active epilepsy to monotherapy with placebo, efficacy of new AEDs is initially tested in placebo-controlled adjunctive therapy (add-on) trials in which patients who are resistant to available treatments [7] are given an experimental treatment or placebo in addition to any therapy on which they are already on. Efficacy is demonstrated when response to the active compound is superior to placebo. As such, the magnitude of placebo response is an important factor in the planning and analysis of clinical trials. A higher than hypothesized placebo response can confound the true treatment effect size. This may result in failure of investigational AEDs to show efficacy. Two large-scale phase III epilepsy trials were recently completed but failed to differentiate drug from placebo, despite having very strong preclinical and preliminary clinical trial evidence of efficacy [1, 24, 25]. An increased variability in the responder rate both across and within studies and, in particular, an observed increased response to placebo with peaks as high as 40% have been noted in several studies [26].

An earlier analysis of randomized controlled trials of adjunctive AEDs showed that response to placebo has increased significantly over time, virtually doubling between 1989 and 2009 [27]. A number of clinical factors were associated with placebo response in patients with refractory focal epilepsy participating in three randomized placebo-controlled trials of lacosamide, a new AED [26]. In multivariate analysis, five factors, which were present prior to the exposure to placebo, were found to be associated with placebo response. Higher age at study entry improved the chances of placebo response. In contrast, a lower chance of placebo response was seen with age at diagnosis of epilepsy of 6–20 years compared to ≤5 years. A history of 7 or more prior lifetime AEDs lowered the chance of achieving placebo response compared to 1–3 prior lifetime AEDs as did a baseline seizure frequency >10 seizures per 28 days compared to ≤5 seizures per 28 days. Prior epilepsy surgery lowered the likelihood of placebo response. This study suggests that a number of prognostic variables may affect placebo response in adults with refractory focal epilepsy [26]. Further studies are needed to assess which prognostic factors that are associated with changes in placebo response are also affecting drug response [7]. Considering and possibly controlling

prognostic factors affecting placebo response may become another challenge in the design of adjunctive AED trials.

Can We Improve Seizure Outcome by Excluding or Adjusting Poor Prognostic Risks?

Employing a strategy to improve seizure outcome by optimizing the proportion of study participants with unfavorable prognostic features will lower the heterogeneity of the sample and result in a larger treatment effect provided that prognostic variables of the controls differ from those of the treatment group. This may mean denying entry to the study for people with poor prognostic features.

A number of possible outcome scenarios when adjusting prognostic variables in randomized AED trials are briefly discussed. A recent study showed that nearly 80% of those meeting the minimum requirement of drug-resistant epilepsy of failure to respond to two suitable AEDs, as defined by the ILAE in 2010, can be expected to achieve 1-year remission [20]. However, restricting trial entry to only those meeting this requirement does not guarantee that an experimental drug is more efficacious than a standard drug or even placebo. The reason is that neither placebo response nor response to a standard AED has been tested in patients meeting the minimum ILAE requirements for drug-resistant epilepsy. Finally, a further limitation is that a positive trial would likely limit the use of the new AED to this restricted patient group and may make it difficult to generalize the finding. This may not favor investment.

Clustering of seizures during treatment, but not prior to treatment, is associated with a poorer long-term seizure and mortality outcome [22]. However, denying entry to patients with a history of seizure clusters during prior AED treatment, does not guarantee a difference in efficacy of the test compound against a standard drug or placebo as placebo response has not been compared in patients with versus no clusters, at least to my knowledge. Finally, a further limitation is that a positive trial in those without a history of clusters, like any other restriction, would likely limit the use of the new AED to a selective patient group and may make it difficult to generalize the finding. This may not favor investment.

Patients with pretreatment seizure frequency of less than once a week and idiopathic or cryptogenic etiology had a threefold higher chance to remain seizure-free from the onset of the first adequate antiepileptic therapy until the end of follow-up compared with patients who had a high pretreatment seizure frequency and a symptomatic etiology [23]. However, denying entry to patients with low pretreatment seizure frequency does not guarantee a difference in efficacy of the test compound against a standard drug or placebo as placebo response has not been compared in patients with versus no clusters (at least to my knowledge). Finally, as with any restriction, this may limit the use of the new AED to a selective patient group and may make it difficult to generalize the finding. This, again, may not favor investment.

Although knowing the predictive factors for the course of epilepsy in the future is informative, the challenge is to translate this insight into clinical benefit. For achieving higher rates of seizure remission on and off AEDs, we may need to eliminate symptomatic causes of epilepsy such as brain injury and the elusive causes of low intelligence. More aggressive treatment early in the course of epilepsy through modern drugs and early evaluation for surgical treatment may prevent children from entering into the dark universe of drug-resistant epilepsy with high morbidity and mortality. One further challenge is to identify factors that predict epileptogenesis, i.e. the underlying disease process that entertains the occurrence of seizures as symptoms [8]. The quest for finding a cure for epilepsy includes a search for predictive factors that drive the development from injury of the brain in the widest sense to the development of the first seizure and, furthermore, what propels the disease to become intractable to drugs and often even to surgery.

Outlook

Current AEDs provide effective antiseizure treatment for the great majority of people with epilepsy: up to 80% become seizure-free on AEDs and 60% remain seizure-free off AEDs. This may explain why new AEDs with traditional or innovative pharmacological mechanisms have not been shown to have better efficacy over available antiseizure treatment. Nevertheless, there is room for improvement. Approximately 20% of people have drug-resistant epilepsy with increased morbidity and mortality compared to the general population and we have no effective treatment to prevent epilepsy or to improve the course of ongoing epilepsy. Longitudinal observations have shown that epilepsy runs in patterns of remission and relapse and that most patients with drug-resistant epilepsy have a neurodeficit and many seizures before or during early AED treatment.

What can we do to further improve the efficacy of antiseizure treatment? We cannot continue to largely imitate traditional antiseizure AEDs and expect change for the better. We need to revolutionize the preclinical and clinical development of AEDs to meet the clinical challenges. Preclinically we need to test new compounds versus standard treatment and explore models to detect efficacy of compounds to prevent epilepsy in those at risk and to change the course and the duration of ongoing epilepsy. Clinical testing needs to explore added benefits in early phase II studies to save costs and provide compelling data to support further investment. Future clinical trial design needs to get away from placebo controls and move to control with standard AEDs and needs to carefully control participants for prognostic features. We need to discover biomarkers that predict poor seizure outcome and high morbidity risk.

References

1 Löscher W, Klitgaard H, Twyman RE, Schmidt D: New avenues for anti-epileptic drug discovery and development. Nat Rev Drug Discov 2013;12:757–776.
2 Löscher W, Schmidt D: Modern antiepileptic drug development has failed to deliver: ways out of the current dilemma. Epilepsia 2011;52:657–678.
3 Sillanpää M, Schmidt D: Natural history of treated childhood-onset epilepsy: Prospective, long-term population-based study. Brain 2006;129:617–624.
4 Shorvon SD, Goodridge DM: Longitudinal cohort studies of the prognosis of epilepsy: contribution of the national general practice study of epilepsy and other studies. Brain 2013;136:3497–3510.
5 Brodie MJ, Barry SJ, Bamagous GA, Norrie JD, Kwan P: Patterns of treatment response in newly diagnosed epilepsy. Neurology 2012;78:1548–1554.
6 Geerts A, Brouwer O, Stroink H, van Donselaar C, Peters B, Peeters E, Arts WF: Onset of intractability and its course over time: the Dutch study of epilepsy in childhood. Epilepsia 2012;53:741–751.
7 Friedman D, French JA: Clinical trials for therapeutic assessment of antiepileptic drugs in the 21st century: obstacles and solutions. Lancet Neurol 2012;11:827–834.
8 Schmidt D, Friedman D, Dichter MA: Anti-epileptogenic clinical trial designs in epilepsy: issues and options. Neurotherapeutics 2014;11:401–411.
9 Schmidt D: Is antiepileptogenesis a realistic goal in clinical trials? Concerns and new horizons. Epileptic Disord 2012;14:105–113.
10 Sillanpää M, Saarinen M, Schmidt D: Clinical conditions of long-term cure in childhood-onset epilepsy: a 45-year follow-up study. Epilepsy Behav 2014;37:49–53.
11 Fisher RA, Acevado C, Arzimanoglou A, et al: ILAE official report: a practical clinical definition of epilepsy. Epilepsia 2014;55:475–482.
12 Hauser W: Commentary: ILAE definition of epilepsy. Epilepsia 2014;55:488–490.
13 Annegers JF, Hauser WA, Elveback LR: Remission of seizures and relapse in patients with epilepsy. Epilepsia 1979;20:729–737.
14 Sillanpää M, Schmidt D: Prognosis of seizure recurrence after stopping antiepileptic drugs in seizure-free patients. A long-term population-based study of childhood-onset epilepsy. Epilepsy Behav 2006;8:713–719.
15 Berg AT, Testa TM, Levy SR: Complete remission in nonsyndromic childhood-onset epilepsy. Ann Neurol 2011;70:566–573.
16 Beyenburg S, Stavem K, Schmidt D: Placebo-corrected efficacy of modern antiepileptic drugs for refractory epilepsy: systematic review and meta-analysis. Epilepsia 2010;51:7–26.
17 Schmidt D, Sillanpää M: Evidence-based review on the natural history of the epilepsies. Curr Opin Neurol 2012;25:159–163.
18 Spooner CG, Berkovic SF, Mitchell LA, Wrennall JA, Harvey AS: New-onset temporal lobe epilepsy in children: lesion on MRI predicts poor seizure outcome. Neurology 2006;67:2117–2118.
19 Sillanpää M, Saarinen M, Schmidt D: Long-term risks following first remission in childhood-onset epilepsy. A population-based study. Epilepsy Behav 2012;25:145–149.
20 Sillanpää M, Schmidt D: Is incident drug-resistance of childhood-onset epilepsy reversible? A long-term follow-up study. Brain 2012;135:2256–2262.
21 Kwan P, Arzimanoglou A, Berg AT, et al: Definition of drug resistant epilepsy: consensus proposal by the ad hoc Task Force of the ILAE Commission on Therapeutic Strategies. Epilepsia 2010;51:1069–1077.
22 Sillanpää M, Schmidt D: Seizure clustering during drug treatment affects seizure outcome and mortality of childhood-onset epilepsy. Brain 2008;131:938–944.
23 Sillanpää M, Schmidt D: Early seizure frequency and aetiology predict long-term medical outcome in childhood-onset epilepsy. Brain 2009;132:989–998.
24 Sperling MR, Greenspan A, Cramer JA, et al: Carisbamate as adjunctive treatment of partial onset seizures in adults in two randomized, placebo-controlled trials. Epilepsia 2010;51:333–343.
25 Halford JJ, Ben-Menachem E, Kwan P, et al: A randomized, double-blind, placebo-controlled study of the efficacy, safety, and tolerability of adjunctive carisbamate treatment in patients with partial-onset seizures. Epilepsia 2011;52:816–825.
26 Schmidt D, Beyenburg S, D'Souza J, Stavem K: Clinical features associated with placebo response in refractory focal epilepsy. Epilepsy Behav 2013;27:393–398.
27 Rheims S, Perucca E, Cucherat M, Ryvlin P: Factors determining response to antiepileptic drugs in randomized controlled trials. A systematic review and meta-analysis. Epilepsia 2011;52:219–233.

Dieter Schmidt
Epilepsy Research Group
Goethestrasse 5
DE–14163 Berlin (Germany)
E-Mail dbschmidt@t-online.de

amino acids with putative antigen-mediated properties. The two drugs have been found to reduce the annualized relapse rate by around 30% in several RCTs, with less consistent data on their ability to delay short-term disability progression. More recently, new drugs have been approved for the market: first-line oral drugs (teriflunomide, dimethyl fumarate) and second-line agents (natalizumab, fingolimod, alemtuzumab, mitoxantrone), which are more effective but also raise serious safety concerns. Several algorithms have been developed to guide clinicians in the treatment of MS patients [14].

Given the absence of long-term RCTs studies, two types of studies are particularly suited to study the long-term efficacy of available drugs, and they have been discussed in a recent review [15]: (1) long-term observational studies to assess the long-term effects of the drug, and (2) long-term extension of follow-up periods for patients included in RCTs.

Long-Term Observational Studies
These studies are divided into two groups based on the type of controls. Concurrent cohort studies compare participants who have received an intervention to those who have not during the same period, while historical cohort studies compare outcomes in a group of patients treated when the drug is available to patients from a previous period when the drug was not available. In concurrent cohort studies, selection bias can occur since patients with a more severe disease course are more likely to choose to be treated, creating an unbalanced distribution of disease prognosis between treated and untreated groups. In historical cohort studies, historical controls tend to have a worse prognosis than current patients [16]. This can be due to diagnostic anticipation driven by improvement in technologies (e.g. MRI), improved care of patients over time, an increase in diagnosis of potential cases, or the capacity to diagnose indolent cases of MS. Another potential bias, especially for historical cohort studies, is

represented by the Will Rogers phenomenon, which is an epidemiological paradox for which moving a patient from one group to another raises or lowers the average value in both groups. This bias has been, for example, demonstrated to be valid in the application of different MS criteria, Poser versus McDonald, on the risk of disability progression, showing that patients diagnosed with older criteria were twice as likely to develop disability progression [17]. To partially overcome this issue, one option is to compare treated patients to those from a geographical region in which the drug can hardly be accessed for economic reasons [18]. It is important to note that the type of control group is crucial, as demonstrated by an interesting study from the British Columbia Multiple Sclerosis Database [19]. By comparing IFN-treated relapsing-remitting MS patients with untreated contemporary and historical cohorts, the authors demonstrated that IFN-β increased the rate of disability progression in comparison with concurrent untreated controls (HR: 1.30), while it decreased it when treated patients were compared to historical controls (HR: 0.77), even if either analysis was not significant.

There are several statistical methods to overcome these biases. Onc is to perform multivariate regression analysis adjusting for potential confounding baseline prognostic variables (provided that they are all known). Another approach is to use the propensity score, which has some advantages over multivariate regression models. In the first step, each patient is assigned a propensity score, which calculates the probability of being treated or untreated according to his or her baseline characteristics. This score is calculated using a standard logistic regression model with unbalanced baseline characteristics as covariates. Outcome measures are then adjusted by the propensity score to offer a comparison between treated and untreated patients which accounts for individual differences. This approach has been used by two large studies on MS patients. One study enrolled 1,504 patients and followed them up for

Table 1. Observational studies assessing long-term effects of IFN-β in patients with relapsing-remitting MS [15]

Study	Treatment and control groups	Follow-up	End point	Statistical approach	Result[1]	Potential biases (bias direction)
Trojano et al. [20], 2007	IFN-β (n = 1,103) vs. contemporary untreated (n = 401)	Median 5.7 years	Time from first visit and from date of birth to SPMS and to EDSS score of 4 or 6 points	Multivariate Cox regression model Propensity score adjustment	Highly significant benefit of IFN-β	Selection bias (favors untreated) Immortal time bias (favors treated)
Brown et al. [22], 2007	Before vs. after IFN-β treatment (n = 590)	24-year observation period	Annualized EDSS change	Fixed-effects model to estimate annual EDSS increase per treatment year	Highly significant benefit of IFN-β	Nonlinearity of progression (favors treatment period) Selection bias (favors untreated periods)
Trojano et al. [21], 2009	Early IFN-β (n = 2,260) vs. late IFN-β (n = 310)	Median 4.5 years	Time from IFN-β treatment start and from date of birth to a confirmed 1-point EDSS progression and to EDSS score of 4 or 6 points	Multivariate Cox regression model Propensity score adjustment	Highly significant benefit of IFN-β	Selection bias (favors untreated), reduced by sensitivity analysis
Veugelers et al. [23], 2009	Before vs. after IFN-β availability (n = 1,752)	24-year observation period	Rates of progression from MS onset to EDSS score of 4, 6, or 8 points	Cox proportional hazards model adjusted for patient characteristics Time from onset to first visit as a time-dependent covariate	Highly significant benefit of IFN-β	Will Rogers phenomenon (favors treated)
Shirani et al. [19], 2012	IFN-β (n = 868) vs. contemporary untreated (n = 829) and historically untreated (n = 959)	Median: IFN-β 5.1 years, concurrent controls 4 years, historical controls 10.8 years	Time from IFN-β treatment eligibility to a confirmed and sustained EDSS score of 6 points	Multivariate Cox regression model with IFN-β treatment as a time-varying covariate Propensity score adjustment	Trend of inferiority of IFN-β vs. contemporary untreated Trend of benefit of IFN-β vs. historically untreated	Selection bias (favors treated when compared with historical control groups, but untreated when compared with concurrent control groups)
Bergamaschi et al. [27], 2012	IFN-β or GA (n = 606) vs. contemporary untreated (n = 478)	Median: treated 16.6 years, untreated 18.3 years	Time from diagnosis to conversion to SPMS	Multivariate Cox regression model adjusted for BREMS score	Highly significant effect of IFN-β and GA therapies	Selection bias (favors untreated)
Tedeholm et al. [28], 2013	IFN-β (n = 730) vs. historical untreated (n = 186)	12-year observation period	Time from disease onset to conversion to SPMS	Cox proportional hazards model adjusted for baseline covariates, time from onset to treatment start and 'period' (historical vs. concurrent) effect	Trend of benefit of IFN-β vs. no treatment, lower than the period effect	Selection bias (favors treated)
Drulovic et al. [18], 2013	IFN-β (n = 236) vs. concurrent untreated (n = 183)	7-year observation period	Time from disease onset to SPMS and EDSS score of 4 or 6 points	Cox proportional hazards model adjusted for the number of previous relapses	Highly significant benefit of IFN-β	Selection bias (favors untreated), mitigated by unavailability of treatment for untreated

BREMS = Bayesian Risk Estimate for Multiple Sclerosis; GA = glatiramer acetate; SPMS = secondary progressive MS. [1] Highly significant refers to p < 0.01, and consistent results across sensitivity analyses.

a median of 5.7 years, comparing treated and untreated cohorts [20], while the second study compared early versus delayed treatments in 2,570 patients with a median follow-up of 4.5 years [21]. The two studies supported the use of the drug, suggesting a significant effect in reducing the rate of disability progression with hazard ratio reduction ranging from 0.4 to 0.7 using different outcome measures (incidence of conversion into SP, time to EDSS 4.0 and to EDSS 6.0) when compared with untreated patients [20]. However, this approach has been criticized for being subject to the immortal time bias. As a matter of fact, if treated and untreated patients are compared, the day of study entry for treated patients is usually the time of drug start, while for untreated ones it is the time of diagnosis or the time of first admission to the MS center, which is typically before the time of drug start. The time period between diagnosis (or referral to the MS center) and first drug administration corresponds to an immortal time: in this time period, no outcome event could have occurred in the treated cohort because patients with an event would have been included in the untreated group as they reached the outcome while untreated, explaining an inflated rate of early events in the untreated cohort leading to a potential overestimation of the treatment effect. In the second study using the propensity score [21], early treatment significantly reduced the risk of reaching a 1-point progression in EDSS score, with hazard risk reduction of 0.63, and of 0.56 if dealing with the time to reach the EDSS of 4.0. Both studies used sensitivity analysis to adjust for unmeasured confounders.

Another important bias favoring the treated group can occur if analyses do not take into account patients lost to follow-up, since nonresponder patients are more likely to be lost to follow-up than responders. A way to adjust this bias is to perform an intention-to-treat analysis by comparing the treatment groups that includes all patients as originally allocated after randomization. For missing observations, the last value carried forward is the recommended method, in which, for each individual, missing values are replaced by the *last observed* value of that variable. However, this approach is limited by the fact that the last observation does not always reflect the functional status at the time of patients dropout, which is frequently motivated by a relapse or adverse treatment effects. This is different to the per protocol analysis, which is a comparison of treatment groups that includes only those patients who completed the treatment originally allocated.

Another approach is to compare disease course before and after treatment. Results of two studies from the Dalhousie Multiple Sclerosis Research Unit database in Canada [22, 23] showed a significant decrease in the yearly decrease of EDSS score (from 0.16 EDSS points/year to 0.02 points/year after drug start with IFN). This approach has the advantage of performing analyses on same subjects, but it assumes that the rate of disability progression is constant over the course of the disease and that the efficacy of the drug is independent from the time and age in which it is started. In table 1 a general overview of these types of studies is presented.

Long-Term Extension RCTs
In these studies, patients are contacted for participation after the end of an RCT. After the double-blind phase of the study, patients treated with placebo are switched to the active drug, and the only question that can be assessed is the effect of an early treatment (active drug treated) versus a delayed treatment (placebo treated switched to the active drug). A potential source of bias is represented by the informative censoring, which is due to the fact that patients doing poorly while on-treatment are more likely to drop out than patients doing well. If dropout patients are lost to follow-up, and this phenomenon happens more in one group than in the other, results are potentially flawed. This type of bias is more relevant now in light of the many alternative drugs

Table 2. Long-term extension of RCTs of IFN-β in patients with relapsing-remitting MS [15]

Trial	Number analyzed/ enrolled (retention fraction)	Treatment	Follow-up, years	End point	Results (early vs. delayed treatment with IFN-β)
IFN-β Multiple Sclerosis Study Group					
Goodin et al. [24], 2012	366/372 (98%)	IFN-β-1b	21	Time to death	Significant reduction in all-cause mortality (HR 0.52, p = 0.01)
Ebers et al. [25], 2010	260/372 (70%)	IFN-β-1b	16	EDSS milestones	No differences in proportion of patients with EDSS ≥6 points (46% early-treated patients vs. 46% delayed) Deaths not analyzed
Multiple Sclerosis Collaborative Research Group (MSCRG)					
Bermel et al. [29], 2010	136/172 (79%)	IFN-β-1a	15	Self-reported 1-point EDSS progression Other EDSS milestones	Significant benefits or early vs. delayed treatment Mean EDSS scores: 5.1. vs. 5.7 points EDSS change from baseline 2.9 vs. 3.3 points Nonsignificant trends toward benefits or early vs. delayed treatment EDSS progression to 4 points: 73.9 vs. 79.1% EDSS progression to 6 points: 47.8 vs. 58.2% EDSS progression to 7 points: 24.6 vs. 31.3% Median time to death: 12.4 vs. 6.9 years
Rudick et al. [30], 2005	160/172 (93%)	IFN-β-1a	8	Proportion of patients with EDSS score ≥6 points	Progression to 6 points on EDSS 29.1% early vs. 42.0% delayed (p = 0.09)
Prevention of Relapses and Disability by IFN-β-1a Subcutaneously in Multiple Sclerosis (PRISMS)					
Kappos et al. [31], 2006	382/560 (68%)	IFN-β-1a	8	1-point EDSS progression Other EDSS milestones	Proportion progressing after early or delayed treatment depends on how dropouts are counted Dropouts excluded: 60% progression in early-treatment vs. 68% in delayed-treatment groups (p = 0.012) Dropouts counted as progression: 64% early vs. 73% delayed (p = 0.007) Dropouts counted as no progression: 54% early vs. 56% delayed (p = 0.12)

All studies compared treatments with placebo.

available on the market to treat MS patients. To avoid this bias, it is important to look at the proportion of originally enrolled patients who are maintained in the extension study, which is called the retention fraction of the study and represents an important measure of the quality of the study. If a patient drops out, applicable statistical techniques are to perform sensitivity analyses comparing results when assigning dropouts to the group doing worse (worst-case scenario), to the group doing better (best-case scenario), or to either groups (likely scenario). You can see an example of long-term extension studies in table 2, in which long-term studies are described on re-

sponse to IFN-β. As can be seen from the table, the retention fraction ranges from 68 to 98%, and follow-up ranges from 8 to 21 years. The study with the longest follow-up of 21 years [24] explored the impact of the drug on mortality (time to death), showing a significant reduction in all-cause mortality (HR: 0.52, p = 0.01) among 372 IFN-β-1b-treated patients. This outcome, compared to EDSS-based outcomes, is less prone to recall bias, also called response bias. All the other 5 studies (table 2), apart from the one conducted by Ebers et al. [25], found a difference in the proportion of patients who had a disease progression in early versus delayed treatment with IFN-β-1b and IFN-β-1a using different EDSS milestones such as the EDSS change from baseline, the proportion of patients with progression to 4.0, 6.0, and 8.0 on the EDSS scale, and the 1-point EDSS progression.

Using a similar approach, a more recent study [26] analyzed patients who received standard natalizumab treatment in a 6-year follow-up analysis: 196 (61.6%) continued the treatment while 122 (38.4%) had to discontinue it after a median time of 3.5 years for detection of JCV positivity. Patients in the discontinuing group had a more than twofold increased risk of disability worsening (p = 0.007), and a 68% decreased likelihood of experiencing disability reduction (p = 0.009) compared with the continuing group, which poses the question of whether it is appropriate or not

to interrupt the treatment in light of the risk of serious adverse events like the occurrence of progressive multifocal leukoencephalopathy. In this regard, it is extremely important to identify biomarkers which could help to stratify patients based on their risk-benefit profile. A good example is represented by the measurement of antibody titers against JCV before starting natalizumab, which aid to stratify MS patients at risk or not of developing progressive multifocal leukoencephalopathy along the treatment period.

In conclusion, there is an urgent need for long-term studies aimed to assess the long-term efficacy of established disease-modifying drugs for MS. It is even more urgent that these studies be well designed, taking into account the several potential biases that could occur.

References

1 Scalfari A, Knappertz V, Cutter G, Goodin DS, Ashton R, Ebers GC: Mortality in patients with multiple sclerosis. Neurology 2013;81:184–192.
2 Polman CH, Reingold SC, Banwell B, et al: Diagnostic criteria for multiple sclerosis: 2010 revisions to the McDonald criteria. Ann Neurol 2011;69:292–302.
3 Lublin FD, Reingold SC: Defining the clinical course of multiple sclerosis: results of an international survey. National Multiple Sclerosis Society (USA) Advisory Committee on Clinical Trials of New Agents in Multiple Sclerosis. Neurology 1996;46:907–911.
4 Lublin FD, Reingold SC, Cohen JA, et al: Defining the clinical course of multiple sclerosis: the 2013 revisions. Neurology 2014;83:278–286.
5 Confavreux C, Vukusic S: Age at disability milestones in multiple sclerosis. Brain 2006;129:595–605.
6 Kurtzke JF: A new scale for evaluating disability in multiple sclerosis. Neurology 1995;5:580–583.
7 Amato MP, Ponziani G: Quantification of impairment in MS: discussion of the scales in use. Mult Scler 1999;5:216–219.

8 Willoughby EW, Paty DW: Scales for rating impairment in multiple sclerosis: a critique. Neurology 1988;38:1793–1798.
9 Noseworthy JH, Vandervoort MK, Hopkins M, Ebers GC: A referendum on clinical trial research in multiple sclerosis: the opinion of the participants at the Jekyll Island workshop. Neurology 1989;39:977–981.
10 Scalfari A, Neuhaus A, Daumer M, et al: Early relapses, onset of progression, and late outcome in multiple sclerosis. JAMA Neurol 2013;70:214–222.
11 Interferon beta-1b is effective in relapsing-remitting multiple sclerosis. I. Clinical results of a multicenter, randomized, double-blind, placebo-controlled trial. The IFNB Multiple Sclerosis Study Group Neurology 1993;43:655–661.
12 Jacobs LD, Cookfair DL, Rudick RA, et al: Intramuscular interferon beta-1a for disease progression in relapsing multiple sclerosis. Ann Neurol 1996;39:285–294.
13 Randomised double-blind placebo-controlled study of interferon beta-1a in relapsing/remitting multiple sclerosis. PRISMS (Prevention of Relapses and Disability by Interferon beta-1a Subcutaneously in Multiple Sclerosis) Study Group. Lancet 1998;352:1498–1504.

14 Sorensen PS: New management algorithms in multiple sclerosis. Curr Opin Neurol 2014;27:246–259.
15 Sormani MP, Bruzzi P: Can we measure long-term treatment effects in multiple sclerosis? Nat Rev Neurol 2015;11:176–182.
16 Inusah S, Sormani MP, Cofield SS, et al: Assessing changes in relapse rates in multiple sclerosis. Mult Scler 2010;16:1414–1421.
17 Sormani MP, Tintorè M, Rovaris M, et al: Will Rogers phenomenon in multiple sclerosis. Ann Neurol 2008;64:428–433.
18 Drulovic J, Kostic J, Mesaros S, et al: Interferon-beta and disability progression in relapsing-remitting multiple sclerosis. Clin Neurol Neurosurg 2013;115(suppl 1):S65–S69.
19 Shirani A, Zhao Y, Karim ME, et al: Association between use of interferon beta and progression of disability in patients with relapsing-remitting multiple sclerosis. JAMA 2012;308:247–256.
20 Trojano M, Pellegrini F, Fuiani A, et al: New natural history of interferon-β-treated relapsing multiple sclerosis. Ann Neurol 2007;61:300–306.

21 Trojano M, Pellegrini F, Paolicelli D, et al: Real-life impact of early interferon beta therapy in relapsing multiple sclerosis. Ann Neurol 2009;66:513–520.

22 Brown MG, Kirby S, Skedgel C, et al: How effective are disease-modifying drugs in delaying progression in relapsing-onset MS? Neurology 2007;69:1498–1507.

23 Veugelers PJ, Fisk JD, Brown MG, et al: Disease progression among multiple sclerosis patients before and during a disease-modifying drug program: a longitudinal population-based evaluation. Mult Scler 2009;15:1286–1294.

24 Goodin DS, Reder AT, Ebers GC, et al: Survival in MS: a randomized cohort study 21 years after the start of the pivotal IFNβ-1b trial. Neurology 2012;78:1315–1322.

25 Ebers GC, Traboulsee A, Li D, et al: Analysis of clinical outcomes according to original treatment groups 16 years after the pivotal IFNB-1b trial. J Neurol Neurosurg Psychiatry 2010;81:907–912.

26 Prosperini L, Annovazzi P, Capobianco M, et al: Natalizumab discontinuation in patients with multiple sclerosis: profiling risk and benefits at therapeutic crossroads. Mult Scler 2015;21:1713–1722.

27 Bergamaschi R, Quaglini S, Tavazzi E, Amato MP, Paolicelli D, Zipoli V, Romani A, Tortorella C, Portaccio E, D'Onghia M, Garberi F, Bargiggia V, Trojano M: Immunomodulatory therapies delay disease progression in multiple sclerosis. Mult Scler 2012, Epub ahead of print.

28 Tedeholm H, Lycke J, Skoog B, et al: Time to secondary progression in patients with multiple sclerosis treated with first generation immunomodulating drugs. Mult Scler 2013;19:765–774.

29 Bermel RA, Weinstock-Guttman B, Bourdette D, et al: Intramuscular interferon beta-1a therapy in patients with relapsing-remitting multiple sclerosis: a 15-year follow-up study. Mult Scler 2010;16:588–596.

30 Rudick RA, Cutter GR, Baier M, et al: Estimating long-term effects of disease modifying drug therapy in multiple sclerosis. Mult Scler 2005;11:626–634.

31 Kappos L, Traboulsee A, Constantinescu C, et al: Long-term subcutaneous interferon beta-1a therapy in patients with relapsing-remitting MS. Neurology 2006;67:944–953.

Filippo Martinelli Boneschi, PhD
Laboratory of Human Genetics of Neurological Disorders
Department of Neurology and Neurorehabilitation
Institute of Experimental Neurology (INSPE), San Raffaele Scientific Institute
Via Olgettina 48, IT–20132 Milan (Italy)
E-Mail martinelli.filippo@hsr.it

Beghi E, Logroscino G (eds): The Right Therapy for Neurological Disorders. From Randomized Trials to Clinical Practice.
Front Neurol Neurosci. Basel, Karger, 2016, vol 39, pp 101–108 (DOI: 10.1159/000445419)

Biomarkers in Randomized Clinical Trials: Magnetic Resonance Imaging

Jennifer L. Whitwell

Mayo Clinic, Rochester, Minn., USA

Abstract

Background: It is essential that randomized clinical trials (RCTs) incorporate biomarkers of disease progression that would be sensitive to the effects of disease-modifying treatments. Magnetic resonance imaging (MRI) can be safely repeated over time, and is routinely performed in clinical centers, making it an ideal modality to be incorporated into RCTs. ***Summary:*** This chapter discusses potential structural MRI biomarkers that have been proposed for a number of different neurodegenerative disorders, including Alzheimer's disease (AD), dementia with Lewy bodies (DLB), frontotemporal dementia (FTD), progressive supranuclear palsy syndrome (PSPS), and Parkinson's disease (PD). All of these disorders represent targets for ongoing and future RCTs. Rates of hippocampal atrophy and ventricular expansion provide excellent biomarkers of disease progression in AD, and may also provide biomarkers in prodromal and preclinical phases of the disease, as well as in DLB. Rates of ventricular expansion also perform well in FTD, although regional frontal and temporal measurements could also be useful. Rates of midbrain atrophy provide the most feasible MRI biomarker in PSPS. In contrast, PD is not associated with specific patterns of cerebral atrophy and further work is needed in order to define useful MRI biomarkers. Sample size calculations using these MRI biomarkers are presented and discussed. ***Key Messages:*** Rates of cerebral atrophy provide valuable potential biomarkers of disease progression in neurodegenerative disorders, and have already begun to be utilized as outcome measures in RCTs. Measurements from other structural and functional MRI modalities require more longitudinal validation, but may prove to be useful in the future.

© 2016 S. Karger AG, Basel

Magnetic resonance imaging (MRI) is an essential tool in the clinical assessment of neurodegenerative diseases, primarily to rule out possible treatable causes of impairment, but also to aid clinical diagnosis. Measurements from MRI also hold promise as important biomarkers of disease progression for randomized clinical trials (RCTs) in a number of different neurodegenerative diseases. MRI is a low-risk imaging modality that can be safely repeated over time without the need for injection of radioactive ligands, and is routinely performed in clinical centers around the world, making it an ideal modality to be incorporated into RCTs. Measurements from MRI also have advantages over clinical scales in that they are not subjective, not affected by symptomatic benefits of the drug, and not affected by floor and ceiling effects like many clinical scales. However, disadvantages include the fact that MRI cannot be performed in people with certain contraindications such as metal implants or pace makers, or in those who suffer from claustrophobia, and MRI can suffer from artifacts such as motion artifacts that can occur in elderly patients with neurodegenerative disease. Also, measurements from MRI can differ across different MRI sequences and scanner field strengths. Careful scanner calibration is required to ensure longitudinal accuracy.

In order to be considered a potential biomarker for RCTs, MRI metrics should ideally provide an indicator of the underlying pathological process and it should be associated with disease progression and sensitive to small changes in disease progression. In order to demonstrate the association with disease progression, longitudinal study designs are necessary, with change or rate measures, rather than cross-sectional measurements, providing the ideal biomarkers. The biomarkers should also be relatively quick and easy to measure in order to allow the assessment of a large number of scans, and should be able to be measured with high precision over serial MRI and across different centers. An important standard by which biomarkers are judged is the sample size required to power RCTs, with good biomarkers providing lower sample size estimates over short time intervals to ultimately reduce the cost and time required for the trial.

This chapter will discuss longitudinal MRI metrics that have been proposed as potential disease biomarkers across a number of different neurodegenerative diseases, including Alzheimer's disease (AD) [1], dementia with Lewy bodies (DLB) [2], frontotemporal dementia (FTD) [3], progressive supranuclear palsy syndrome (PSPS) [4], and Parkinson's disease (PD) [5], all of which are currently being targeted by RCTs.

Alzheimer's Disease

AD [1] is the most common form of neurodegenerative dementia and hence has been the focus of many studies searching for reliable disease biomarkers. Biomarkers measured from MRI are well suited to AD because it is associated with a well-defined and characteristic pattern of neurodegeneration that can be visualized on structural MRI. Typical late-onset AD is associated with early and striking atrophy of the hippocampi, with additional involvement of the temporal and parietal cortices, and concurrent expansion of the ventricles (fig. 1). Atrophy of these regions in AD appears to reflect an underlying deposition of the protein tau in the brain. Some of the simplest to measure and most effective potential biomarkers are rates of atrophy of the hippocampus or global measures, such as rate of whole brain atrophy or rate of expansion of the ventricles [6–10]. Longitudinal studies have shown that these rate measures are increased in AD compared to healthy controls and correlate well with cognitive decline over time. Studies have shown that these measures provide reasonable sample size estimates for RCTs, with sample sizes reported between 75 and 150 subjects required per arm to power a 12-month RCT (table 1). Variability in reported estimates depends in a large part on the predicted treatment effect and the power of the study. Rates of hippocampal and whole brain atrophy, and ventricular expansion have, in fact, already been employed as biomarkers in a number of RCTs in AD.

Measurements of other regional structures also hold promise as potential biomarkers in AD, with some studies finding optimal sample size estimates with rates of atrophy of the entorhinal cortex [11] or temporal lobe [12]. Methodological optimizations and enhancements may also help reduce sample size estimates [13]; however, with greater technical specification, biomarkers run the risk of being more difficult to implement across centers with varying technical capabilities.

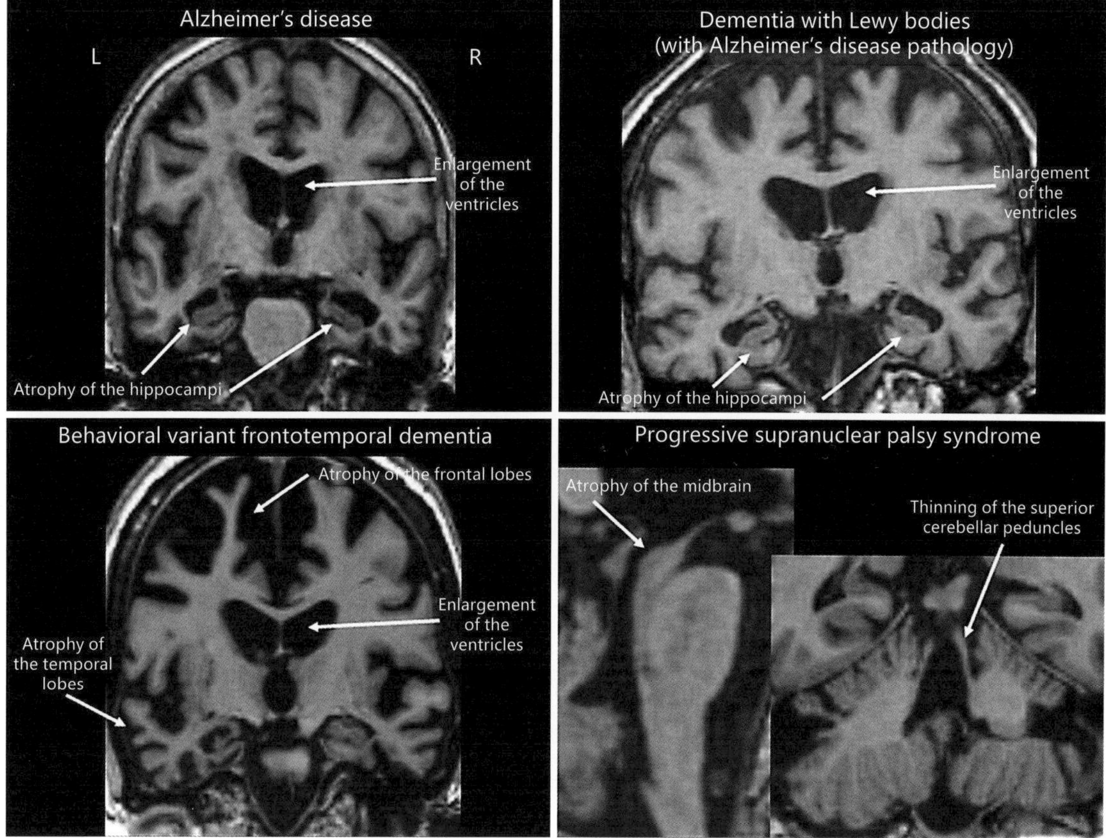

Fig. 1. Structural MRI illustrating the signature patterns of brain atrophy and ventricular expansion in four neurodegenerative disorders.

There is also evidence that sample size estimates can be reduced by accounting for other factors, such as the presence of the apolipoprotein ε4 allele [10, 12], a risk factor for AD, or by increasing the length of the RCT to 24 months [12]. The Alzheimer's Disease Neuroimaging Initiative (ADNI; http://www.adni-info.org), a large multisite longitudinal study on AD, was in fact set up primarily with the goal of investigating optimal biomarkers for RCTs. Subjects in the first cycle of ADNI were followed every 6 months for 24 months, and a number of studies have reported excellent sample size estimates utilizing the 24-month data, with sample size estimates reduced by approximately 30% compared to the 12-month estimates (table 1). Some studies have also investigated the value of MRI biomarkers for a 6-month RCT, although sample size estimates over this period were, understandably, much larger than those reported at 12 months (table 1), largely due to increased measurement error over short intervals [8]. Regardless of the interval assessed or specific method utilized, MRI biomarkers strongly outperform clinical biomarkers [10, 11].

There has also been an increasing emphasis on being able to identify patients with AD early in their disease course since treatments for AD are most likely to be effective before patients become demented. Patients in the prodromal stage of AD,

Table 1. MRI biomarker sample size estimates from a selection of studies assessing different neurodegenerative diseases

Reference	Population	n	Scan interval, months	MRI rate measure	Treatment effect, %	Power, %	Estimated sample size
Fox et al. [6], 2000	AD	18	12	Whole brain	20	90	115 or 168[a]
Jack et al. [7], 2003	AD	192	12	Hippocampal	50	90	21
Schott et al. [8], 2005	AD	38	12	Ventricular	20	90	141
	AD	38	6	Ventricular	20	90	165
Nestor et al. [9], 2008[b]	AD	105	6	Ventricular	20	90	342
	MCI	247	6	Ventricular	20	90	1,180
Schuff et al. [10], 2009[b]	AD	96	12	Hippocampal	25	90	252
	MCI	226	12	Hippocampal	25	90	698
	AD	96	6	Hippocampal	25	90	462
	MCI	226	6	Hippocampal	25	90	949
Holland et al. [11], 2009[b]	AD	129	24	Entorhinal	25	80	45 or 65[a]
	MCI	299	24	Entorhinal	25	80	135 or 241[a]
Holland et al. [15], 2012[b]	MCI (Aβ+, ptau+, MRI+)	71	36	Entorhinal	25	80	60[a]
	CN (Aβ+, ptau+)	21	36	Amygdala	25	80	773
Hua et al. [12], 2013[b]	AD	188	12	Temporal lobe	25	80	58
	MCI	400	12	Temporal lobe	25	80	124
	AD	188	24	Temporal lobe	25	80	39
	MCI	400	24	Temporal lobe	25	80	95
Gutman et al. [13], 2013[b]	AD	144	12	Ventricular	25	80	75
	MCI	337	12	Ventricular	25	80	104
	AD	111	24	Ventricular	25	80	52
	MCI	253	24	Ventricular	25	80	67
Andrews et al. [14], 2013	CN (Aβ+)	22	18	Hippocampal	25	80	384
Nedelska et al. [18], 2015	DLB/AD	22	12	Ventricular	25	80	43
Rohrer et al. [24], 2008	SD	21	12	Temporal lobe	30	90	44 or 55[a]
Knopman et al. [23], 2009	bvFTD	34	12	Ventricular	25	80	127
	agPPA	17	12	Ventricular	25	80	55
	SD	16	12	Ventricular	25	80	58
Paviour et al. [26], 2007	PSPS	17	12	Midbrain	30	90	147[a]
Whitwell et al. [25], 2012	PSPS	16	6	Midbrain	30	90	262[a]
	PSPS	16	12	Midbrain	30	90	84[a]

Sample sizes are shown for the optimal MRI biomarker obtained in each study. Aβ+ = Evidence of β-amyloid deposition on positron emission tomography; agPPA = agrammatic variant of primary progressive aphasia; bvFTD = behavioral variant FTD; CN = cognitively normal; CSF = cerebrospinal fluid; MRI+ = evidence of atrophy on MRI; ptau+ = elevated hyperphosphorylated tau measured from CSF; SD = semantic dementia. [a] Sample size estimates accounting for normal aging. [b] Data from the ADNI.

known as mild cognitive impairment (MCI), typically show increased rates of hippocampal and temporal atrophy compared to healthy controls, although the rates are lower than those observed in AD. Biomarkers that have been developed for AD are therefore also largely applicable to MCI, with reasonable sample size estimates obtained in MCI cohorts (table 1). There is some evidence that the required sample size can be further reduced if a trial was enriched and only recruited

MCI patients with evidence of β-amyloid deposition on positron emission tomography (PET) imaging, elevated hyperphosphorylated tau in cerebrospinal fluid, and evidence of atrophy on MRI. This process of enrichment increases the chance that MCI patients do indeed have underlying AD pathology and are on the path to developing AD. It may, however, be possible to identify subjects in preclinical stages of the disease, before the occurrence of any symptoms.

Approximately one third of cognitively normal elderly people have evidence of β-amyloid deposition on PET scanning, suggesting that they may have underlying AD pathology. Although little is currently known about the fate of these people, there is some evidence that they may show increased rates of hippocampal atrophy compared to cognitively normal people that do not have β-amyloid deposition on PET [14]. However, sample sizes needed to power RCTs using these preclinical subjects are large, ranging between 384 and 773 subjects required per arm [14, 15] (table 1). These sample sizes may, however, be achievable given that cognitively normal elderly people may be easier to enroll than patients that already have a neurodegenerative disease. A secondary prevention trial has, in fact, already begun using this population (http://a4study.org). Another potential target for assessing preclinical AD is to recruit cognitively normal people that have autosomal dominant AD mutations. Increased rates of hippocampal atrophy can be observed in these subjects 5 years before they become symptomatic, suggesting that MRI biomarkers could be fruitful for RCTs focusing on this population.

Dementia with Lewy Bodies

DLB [2] is the second most common dementia in the elderly [16]. It is associated primarily with α-synuclein pathology, although a large number of subjects also have coexistent AD pathologies.

Progressive brain atrophy is a feature of DLB, although this is typically observed in subjects who also have underlying AD pathologies [17]. Rates of whole brain and hippocampal atrophy are increased in subjects with mixed DLB and AD pathologies compared to healthy controls, with rates associated with the severity of underlying tau pathology [17, 18]. Rates of atrophy in subjects with pure DLB are no different to those reported in healthy controls [17, 18]. Rates of ventricular expansion appear to provide the optimum sample size estimates in subjects with mixed DLB and AD, so they may be useful as biomarkers of AD pathology in these subjects [18] (table 1). The reason that ventricular measures often provide excellent sample size is likely because they can be measured with a high degree of accuracy and are often less affected by scan artifacts than other regional or global measures. Future RCTs aiming to utilize these MRI biomarkers will need to recruit patients who have mixed DLB and AD pathologies, perhaps with the aid of β-amyloid PET scanning. It will be hard to determine clinically whether a patient diagnosed with DLB in fact has mixed underlying pathologies.

Frontotemporal Dementia

FTD [3] is as common as AD in people under the age of 65 years [19]. The umbrella term of FTD has been used to capture three main clinical syndromes, behavioral variant FTD [20], semantic dementia [21], and agrammatic/nonfluent primary progressive aphasia [21], which are each associated with focal lobar atrophy affecting the frontal and temporal lobes (fig. 1). Rates of whole brain atrophy and ventricular expansion are typically increased in all three of these FTD syndromes compared to healthy controls, and are also increased compared to subjects with AD [22]. These measures, particularly rate of ventricular expansion, are therefore promising biomarkers for these syndromes, and provide small sample size estimates for RCTs [23] (table 1). However, given the focal nature of degeneration in the FTD syndromes, regional MRI measures may provide better biomarkers. For example, rate of temporal lobe atrophy gives higher rates of atrophy and better sample size estimates in semantic dementia compared to whole brain measures [24] (table 1).

A number of genetic mutations have been shown to cause familial FTD, including mutations in the microtubule-associated protein tau and progranulin genes, and repeat expansions in C9ORF72. Rate of ventricular expansion has provided excellent sample size estimates of 191 subjects for microtubule-associated protein tau, 61 subjects for progranulin, and 56 subjects for C9ORF72 per treatment arm to detect a 20% treatment effect at 80% power (unpubl. data). Similar MRI biomarkers could, therefore, be utilized both in sporadic and familial forms of FTD. In addition, these genetic mutations provide the possibility that future RCTs could target asymptomatic mutation carriers to allow early treatment benefits. There is, indeed, some evidence that atrophy can be detected before symptom onset in mutation carriers.

Progressive Supranuclear Palsy Syndrome

PSPS [4] is a movement disorder which has a close clinicopathological association with underlying tau pathology. It is a devastating disorder which has been the focus of many RCTs, particularly those evaluating therapies aimed at targeting tau. It is hoped that disease-modifying therapies that can target tau in PSPS may also prove to be beneficial in other disorders that have tau deposition, such as AD. It is therefore crucial that appropriate outcome measures are available for use in this cohort.

An advantage of targeting PSPS is that it is associated with characteristic patterns of atrophy which can be detected on MRI, including atrophy of the midbrain, superior cerebellar peduncles, and premotor cortex (fig. 1). Increased rates of atrophy can be detected in these regions over a 12-month interval, with increased rates of midbrain atrophy also detectable over 6 months [25]. Rates of atrophy also correlate well with clinical disease progression. Optimal sample size estimates in PSPS have been obtained using rate of midbrain atrophy, with only 84 subjects required per arm to provide power to detect a 30% treatment effect [25] (table 1). These sample size estimates are smaller than those obtained with rates of whole brain atrophy or ventricular expansion [25, 26], and are also smaller than those obtained using a clinical severity scale (the PSP rating scale) [25], suggesting that a regional measurement of the midbrain is the most feasible MRI biomarker for PSPS. Importantly, it can also be measured using automated methods and would therefore be a relatively quick and easy measure to apply in an RCT. Sample size estimates obtained with rate of whole brain atrophy and ventricular expansion were, however, still reasonable in PSPS [25]; therefore, these measures could be feasible biomarker additions to an RCT. MRI biomarkers have already been employed in RCTs of PSPS, with one trial demonstrating that the drug tideglusib can slow the rate of regional and whole brain atrophy in PSPS over 12 months with only 37 subjects [27].

Parkinson's Disease

In contrast to the other neurodegenerative disorders discussed above, PD [5] is not associated with a clear pattern of neurodegeneration on MRI. There is some evidence that rates of brain atrophy are increased in subjects with PD, particularly in subjects that also have MCI or dementia [28], but these rates do not seem to correlate to clinical measures of disease severity and the findings have not been corroborated by any other studies. It is, therefore, unclear whether there are any appropriate structural

MRI biomarkers of disease progression that could be useful for RCTs in PD. MRI techniques that allow better visualization of the nigrostriatal system, measurement of iron load in the brain, or measurement of diffusivity in the nigrostriatal system [29] could have potential, but a lot more work is needed to determine the feasibility of these methods for longitudinal measurement. Currently, functional neuroimaging methods, including PET and single-photon emission computed tomography, hold greater promise as potential disease biomarkers in PD.

Conclusions and Future Directions

MRI biomarkers have been shown to be feasible outcome measures for RCTs across a range of different neurodegenerative disorders. These biomarkers will be invaluable with the advent of potential disease-modifying treatments. Structural biomarkers, particularly rates of brain atrophy, have received the most attention, with regional measurements targeted to the specific disorder often providing optimum sample size estimates for trials and outperforming clinical measures. However, many of these MRI studies suffer from limitations that should be considered, such as not accounting for potential patient dropout, not calculating sample sizes using the excess change over normal aging, and not incorporating multisite MRI data. Failing to account for these variables could produce unrealistically low sample size estimates.

A number of other MRI modalities may also produce useful disease biomarkers in the future, such as diffusion tensor imaging which allows the assessment of white matter tract integrity, task-free functional MRI which assesses functional connectivity within the brain, and arterial spin labelling which measures cerebral blood flow. These modalities have shown promising results in cross-sectional studies across these neurodegenerative diseases, but need further validation in longitudinal studies before they can be utilized in future RCTs.

References

1 McKhann GM, Knopman DS, Chertkow H, et al: The diagnosis of dementia due to Alzheimer's disease: recommendations from the National Institute on Aging-Alzheimer's Association workgroups on diagnostic guidelines for Alzheimer's disease. Alzheimers Dement 2011;7:263–269.

2 McKeith IG, Dickson DW, Lowe J, et al: Diagnosis and management of dementia with Lewy bodies: third report of the DLB Consortium. Neurology 2005;65:1863–1872.

3 Neary D, Snowden JS, Gustafson L, et al: Frontotemporal lobar degeneration: a consensus on clinical diagnostic criteria. Neurology 1998;51:1546–1554.

4 Litvan I, Agid Y, Calne D, et al: Clinical research criteria for the diagnosis of progressive supranuclear palsy (Steele-Richardson-Olszewski syndrome): report of the NINDS-SPSP international workshop. Neurology 1996;47:1–9.

5 Hughes AJ, Daniel SE, Kilford L, Lees AJ: Accuracy of clinical diagnosis of idiopathic Parkinson's disease: a clinicopathological study of 100 cases. J Neurol Neurosurg Psychiatry 1992;55:181–184.

6 Fox NC, Cousens S, Scahill R, Harvey RJ, Rossor MN: Using serial registered brain magnetic resonance imaging to measure disease progression in Alzheimer disease: power calculations and estimates of sample size to detect treatment effects. Arch Neurol 2000;57:339–344.

7 Jack CR Jr, Slomkowski M, Gracon S, et al: MRI as a biomarker of disease progression in a therapeutic trial of milameline for AD. Neurology 2003;60:253–260.

8 Schott JM, Price SL, Frost C, Whitwell JL, Rossor MN, Fox NC: Measuring atrophy in Alzheimer disease: a serial MRI study over 6 and 12 months. Neurology 2005;65:119–124.

9 Nestor SM, Rupsingh R, Borrie M, et al: Ventricular enlargement as a possible measure of Alzheimer's disease progression validated using the Alzheimer's disease neuroimaging initiative database. Brain 2008;131:2443–2454.

10 Schuff N, Woerner N, Boreta L, et al: MRI of hippocampal volume loss in early Alzheimer's disease in relation to ApoE genotype and biomarkers. Brain 2009;132:1067–1077.

11 Holland D, Brewer JB, Hagler DJ, Fennema-Notestine C, Dale AM; Alzheimer's Disease Neuroimaging Initiative: Subregional neuroanatomical change as a biomarker for Alzheimer's disease. Proc Natl Acad Sci USA 2009;106:20954–20959.

12 Hua X, Hibar DP, Ching CR, et al: Unbiased tensor-based morphometry: improved robustness and sample size estimates for Alzheimer's disease clinical trials. Neuroimage 2013;66:648–661.

13 Gutman BA, Hua X, Rajagopalan P, et al: Maximizing power to track Alzheimer's disease and MCI progression by LDA-based weighting of longitudinal ventricular surface features. Neuroimage 2013; 70:386–401.

14 Andrews KA, Modat M, Macdonald KE, et al: Atrophy rates in asymptomatic amyloidosis: implications for Alzheimer prevention trials. PLoS One 2013; 8:e58816.

15 Holland D, McEvoy LK, Desikan RS, Dale AM; Alzheimer's Disease Neuroimaging Initiative: Enrichment and stratification for predementia Alzheimer disease clinical trials. PLoS One 2012; 7:e47739.

16 Tola-Arribas MA, Yugueros MI, Garea MJ, et al: Prevalence of dementia and subtypes in Valladolid, northwestern Spain: the DEMINVALL study. PLoS One 2013;8:e77688.

17 Whitwell JL, Jack CR Jr, Parisi JE, et al: Rates of cerebral atrophy differ in different degenerative pathologies. Brain 2007;130:1148–1158.

18 Nedelska Z, Ferman TJ, Boeve BF, et al: Pattern of brain atrophy rates in autopsy-confirmed dementia with Lewy bodies. Neurobiol Aging 2015;36:452–461.

19 Ratnavalli E, Brayne C, Dawson K, Hodges JR: The prevalence of frontotemporal dementia. Neurology 2002;58: 1615–1621.

20 Rascovsky K, Hodges JR, Knopman D, et al: Sensitivity of revised diagnostic criteria for the behavioural variant of frontotemporal dementia. Brain 2011;134: 2456–2477.

21 Gorno-Tempini ML, Hillis AE, Weintraub S, et al: Classification of primary progressive aphasia and its variants. Neurology 2011;76:1006–1014.

22 Whitwell JL, Jack CR Jr, Pankratz VS, et al: Rates of brain atrophy over time in autopsy-proven frontotemporal dementia and Alzheimer disease. Neuroimage 2008;39:1034–1040.

23 Knopman DS, Jack CR Jr, Kramer JH, et al: Brain and ventricular volumetric changes in frontotemporal lobar degeneration over 1 year. Neurology 2009;72: 1843–1849.

24 Rohrer JD, McNaught E, Foster J, et al: Tracking progression in frontotemporal lobar degeneration: serial MRI in semantic dementia. Neurology 2008;71: 1445–1451.

25 Whitwell JL, Xu J, Mandrekar JN, Gunter JL, Jack CR Jr, Josephs KA: Rates of brain atrophy and clinical decline over 6 and 12-month intervals in PSP: determining sample size for treatment trials. Parkinsonism Relat Disord 2012;18: 252–256.

26 Paviour DC, Price SL, Lees AJ, Fox NC: MRI derived brain atrophy in PSP and MSA-P. Determining sample size to detect treatment effects. J Neurol 2007; 254:478–481.

27 Hoglinger GU, Huppertz HJ, Wagenpfeil S, et al: Tideglusib reduces progression of brain atrophy in progressive supranuclear palsy in a randomized trial. Mov Disord 2014;29:479–487.

28 Burton EJ, McKeith IG, Burn DJ, O'Brien JT: Brain atrophy rates in Parkinson's disease with and without dementia using serial magnetic resonance imaging. Mov Disord 2005;20:1571–1576.

29 Pyatigorskaya N, Gallea C, Garcia-Lorenzo D, Vidailhet M, Lehericy S: A review of the use of magnetic resonance imaging in Parkinson's disease. Ther Adv Neurol Disord 2014;7:206–220.

Jennifer L. Whitwell, Associate Professor of Radiology
Mayo Clinic
200 1st St. SW
Rochester, MN 55905 (USA)
E-Mail whitwell.jennifer@mayo.edu

Beghi E, Logroscino G (eds): The Right Therapy for Neurological Disorders. From Randomized Trials to Clinical Practice.
Front Neurol Neurosci. Basel, Karger, 2016, vol 39, pp 109–116 (DOI: 10.1159/000445451)

Biomarkers in Randomized Clinical Trials: Positron Emission Tomography and Nuclear Medicine Techniques

Tarun Singhal[a] · Emily Stern[b, c]

Departments of [a]Neurology, [b]Radiology, and [c]Psychiatry, Brigham and Women's Hospital, Harvard Medical School,
Boston, Mass., USA

Abstract

Background: Positron emission tomography (PET) and
single-photon emission computed tomography (SPECT)
are nuclear medicine techniques that utilize the tracer
principle to image biological processes using radiola-
beled molecules. Numerous PET and SPECT radiopharmaceuticals have been developed over the years that
qualify as biomarkers for neurological disorders. **Summary:** This chapter reviews the use of PET and SPECT in neurological clinical trials, and emphasizes the concepts and
lessons learned from these experiences. **Key Messages:**
Key considerations for successful use of PET or SPECT imaging as biomarkers in neurological randomized trials include: (1) in vivo behavior of the radiotracer and the PET
or SPECT imaging parameter studied should reflect an essential aspect of the underlying pathology and/or pathophysiology of the disease under question, (2) the underlying biological target and radiotracer distribution should
have the potential to vary with treatment under study
conditions, and adjustments must be made for any other
known changes (e.g. physiological) that may occur over
time, (3) image reconstruction techniques and quantitative or semiquantitative image analysis approaches
should be robust and standardized across trial sites, and
(4) newer molecular targets should be explored based on
insights obtained from basic science research and translational observations. Successful implementation of PET
and SPECT in clinical trials and practice has a highly significant potential to contribute towards improving outcomes and clinical care for patients with neurological disorders.

A 'biomarker' has been defined as 'a characteristic
that is objectively measured and evaluated as an
indicator of normal biological processes, pathogenic processes, or pharmacological responses to
a therapeutic intervention' [1, 2]. Positron emission tomography (PET) and single-photon emission computed tomography (SPECT) are nuclear
medicine techniques that utilize the tracer principle to image biological processes using radiola-
beled molecules. These are powerful molecular
imaging tools that provide unique insights into

Table 1. Examples of radiopharmaceuticals used in neurological diseases

Radiopharmaceutical(s)	Biological target	Disease condition/application
[^{11}C]PiB, [^{18}F]florbetapir	β-Amyloid	AD [16]
[^{123}I]β-CIT, [^{123}I]ioflupane	Dopamine transporter	Parkinson's disease [7]
[^{15}O]H$_2$O	Cerebral blood flow	Stroke [19]
[^{11}C]Raclopride	Dopamine (D2) receptor	Dose occupancy studies of antipsychotics [21]
[^{11}C]PK11195	18-kDa translocator protein (TSPO)	Neuroinflammation/microglial activation [21]

PiB = Pittsburgh compound B; CIT = 2β-carbomethoxy-3β-(4-iodophenyl)tropane.

the pathophysiology of various brain disorders and have been demonstrated to be clinically useful in diagnosing and monitoring of several of these conditions [3, 4]. PET and SPECT enable detection of abnormalities earlier in the course of a disease than conventional imaging techniques (e.g. computed tomography and conventional magnetic resonance imaging) because functional and molecular changes detected by PET and SPECT can often precede structural changes targeted by the conventional modalities. PET and SPECT also provide a unique opportunity to directly study biologic processes that may not have an obvious structural imaging correlate at all, such as a wide plethora of neuropsychiatric conditions [5]. In addition to visual qualitative analyses, PET and SPECT are amenable quantitative and semiquantitative estimations of biologically relevant parameters.

For these reasons, a large number of PET and SPECT radiopharmaceuticals have been developed over the years that qualify as biomarkers for neurological disorders (table 1) [6]. They serve as diagnostic, prognostic, and predictive markers, disease activity markers, and as drug effect and drug kinetics biomarkers [1].

This chapter aims to review the use of PET and SPECT in clinical trials of some of the most prevalent neurological disorders, as illustrations of the concepts involved and to subsequently emphasize the lessons thus far learned from these experiences.

Examples of PET and SPECT Imaging in Neurological Clinical Trials

Parkinson's Disease

Parkinson's disease is characterized by loss of dopaminergic neurons arising from the substantia nigra in the midbrain and their projection terminals in the caudate and putamen. Treatment with dopaminergic agents (e.g. levodopa/carbidopa) as well as dopamine agonists (e.g. pramipexole or ropinirole) has been a mainstay of therapy in this condition. While these treatments provide gratifying symptomatic relief, particularly in earlier stages of disease, better treatments are needed that have a definite neuroprotective role and either prevent or slow down the rate of decline in these patients.

Clinical trials in Parkinson's disease, as in other neurodegenerative conditions have an overarching goal to objectively assess neuroprotective therapies as well as to study any neurotoxic effects of existing symptomatic treatments. While clinical assessment has its own advantages and has been formalized through development of several clinical scales, such as the Unified Parkinson's Disease Rating Scale (UPDRS), it may be considered subjective and prone to examiner and examinee bias. In addition, clinical scales may emphasize one clinical feature over another and may not accurately reflect the underlying biological changes. Moreover, symptomatic benefits of treatment may mask the ongoing neurodegeneration when assessed by clinical means alone.

[^{123}I]β-CIT is a tropane analogue SPECT tracer that binds to presynaptic dopamine transporter and has high specific uptake in a normal putamen and caudate. Similarly, [^{18}F-]fluorodopa is a PET tracer that also has presynaptic uptake in the basal ganglia and reflects the enzymatic activity of DOPA decarboxylase in dopaminergic terminals. There is decreased basal ganglia uptake of both tracers in Parkinson's disease that is generally more prominent in the posterior putamen in early disease and subsequently involves the rest of basal ganglia as the disease progresses.

Fahn et al. [7] randomized patients with early Parkinson's disease (n = 361) into three treatment arms receiving different doses of levodopa/carbidopa and one placebo arm for 40 weeks followed by a 2-week 'washout period'. They assessed the clinical severity after the 42 weeks' duration of the trial using UPDRS. They determined that there was a clinical worsening of Parkinson's disease in the placebo arm as compared to the treatment arms (p < 0.001). On the other hand, when the investigators performed a substudy on 116 patients who had a baseline abnormal [^{123}I]β-CIT scan and completed 40 weeks of follow-up, they found a decrease in radiotracer binding in patients receiving levodopa as compared to the placebo arm. Hence, it was inferred that clinical and SPECT imaging revealed opposite results in terms of the effect of levodopa on Parkinson's disease.

The exact reasons for this discrepancy remain unclear. It has been speculated that SPECT scans were performed without any levodopa washout period and that may have interfered with radiotracer binding, contributing to falsely low tracer uptake at the end of 40 weeks of follow-up. However, in routine clinical use, it is not recommended to stop levodopa treatment prior to dopamine transporter imaging, as levodopa is generally not thought to interfere with tracer binding to its target [8].

Moreover, this study had approximately 15% of its subjects had scans without evidence of dopaminergic deficit (SWEDD). Longitudinal follow-up of SWEDD subjects in subsequent studies has demonstrated no evidence of clinical or imaging progression, suggesting that SWEDD subjects are unlikely to have idiopathic Parkinson's disease [9].

In another study, patients with Parkinson's disease were randomized to receive either levodopa/carbidopa or pramipexole and underwent [^{123}I]β-CIT scans at baseline, 22, 34, and 46 months after initiation of treatment. It was demonstrated that the rate of decline of [^{123}I]β-CIT binding was slower for pramipexole versus levodopa. This was interpreted to be a result of either a protective effect of pramipexole or a deleterious effect of levodopa on dopaminergic neurons [10].

The relation between clinical indices and molecular imaging of the dopaminergic system is complex. Several cross-sectional studies have demonstrated a correlation between [^{123}I]β-CIT binding and UPDRS scores, but the correlation between longitudinal changes in UPDRS scores and [^{123}I]β-CIT or [^{18}F]fluorodopa uptake over time has been less consistent [10–14]. Moreover, while [18F]fluorodopa activity has been shown to correlate well with nigral neuron density, [^{18}F-]fluorodopa may underestimate neuronal loss in the early stages of the disease because of a compensatory upregulation of dopa decarboxylase, the enzyme responsible for its retention in dopaminergic nerve terminals. On the other hand, [^{123}I]β-CIT may overestimate neuronal loss because of compensatory downregulation of the dopamine transporter in adjacent neurons. In addition, there is a physiological decline in [^{123}I]β-CIT binding with aging that needs to be adjusted for in longitudinal studies [15]. A fluoropropyl derivative of [^{123}I]β-CIT ([^{123}I]ioflupane or FP-CIT) is available commercially for clinical use (table 1, fig. 1).

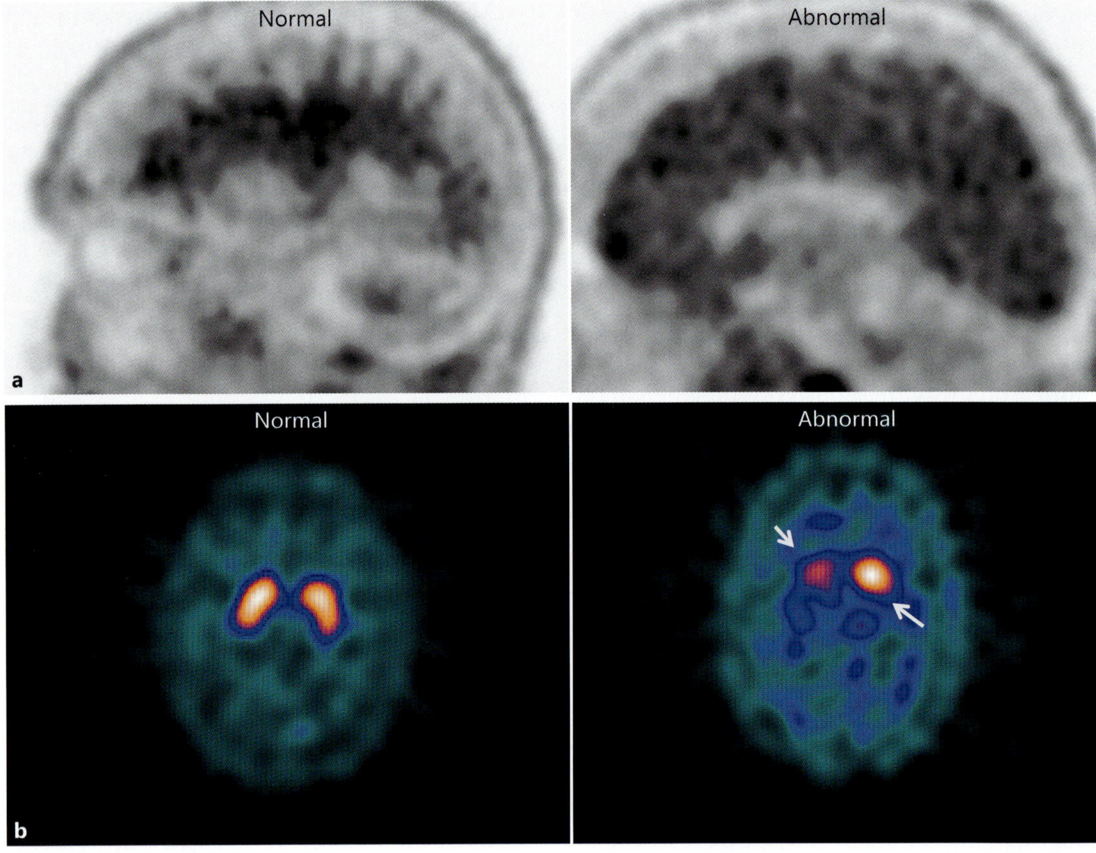

Fig. 1. a [¹⁸F]Florbetapir amyloid PET scan. Sagittal image in a normal scan (left) reveals preserved grey-white matter differentiation while an abnormal scan (right) demonstrates abnormal radiotracer accumulation in the grey matter with a loss of grey-white matter differentiation. **b** [¹²³I]Ioflupane SPECT scan reveals normal tracer accumulation in the bilateral caudate and putamen (left), while an abnormal image shows markedly decreased radiotracer accumulation in the right caudate and bilateral putamen (arrows).

Another pathological hallmark of Parkinson's disease is the presence of intracellular 'Lewy bodies', aggregates of a protein called α-synuclein. Lewy body appearance may precede dopaminergic cell loss by years. Identification of abnormal α-synuclein deposition may hence, provide the earliest detection of Parkinson's disease and longitudinal changes in α-synuclein deposition may better correlate with clinical course than imaging of the dopaminergic system. There is no viable radiotracer yet for imaging of brain α-synuclein [16]. Development of such a radiotracer will fulfill a major unmet need in the field.

Alzheimer's Disease

Alzheimer's disease (AD) is the most common cause of progressive dementia. β-Amyloid deposition in the cerebral cortex is a pathological hallmark of AD. Several [¹¹C]- and [¹⁸F]-labeled PET radiopharmaceuticals have been developed for amyloid imaging, including [¹¹C]PiB, [¹⁸F]florbetapir (fig. 1), [¹⁸F]florbetaben, and [¹⁸F]flutemetamol.

In a phase II placebo-controlled trial, bapineuzumab, a humanized anti-amyloid-β monoclonal antibody was administered to 20 patients with mild-to-moderate AD who underwent [¹¹C]PiB

PET scans at baseline, 20, 45, and 78 weeks [17]. Cortical-to-cerebellar ratios of [^{11}C]PiB retention were measured. At 78 weeks, there was a net decrease in [^{11}C]PiB retention in the treatment arm as compared to baseline and a net increase in the placebo arm (p = 0.014 and 0.022, respectively). In addition, investigators performed in vitro assays with bapineuzumab and [^{3}H]PiB, and determined that bapineuzumab did not compete with [^{3}H]PiB binding in AD brain homogenates or synthetic amyloid-β fibrils [17].

Based on these findings, two phase III trials of bapineuzumab in mild-to-moderate AD were conducted in separate cohorts of apolipoprotein E ε4 allele carriers (n = 1,121) and noncarriers (n = 1,331) [18]. A subset of patients underwent [^{11}C] PiB imaging and those with a standardized uptake value ratio (SUVR) greater than 1.35 (calculated as an average of SUVRs for five cortical areas) were considered to be 'amyloid-positive' and underwent follow-up imaging in both the treatment and placebo arms. Interestingly, approximately 36% of noncarriers as compared to only 6.5% of carriers did not meet the SUVR threshold and were not included in the data analysis.

In terms of changes in [^{11}C]PiB uptake, there was no statistically significant difference between the two groups in the trial performed on noncarriers (n = 39). Among carriers (n = 115), SUVR increased at the 71-week follow-up as compared to baseline in the placebo group (difference in SUVR = 0.102 ± 0.026), but remained almost stable in the bapineuzumab treatment group (difference in SUVR = 0.001 ± 0.021), and the difference in the change between the treatment and placebo groups was statistically significant (p = 0.004). However, in both trials there was no statistically significant change in clinical measures of cognitive status. In addition, no significant changes in brain atrophy measures were seen in any groups in both trials. Cerebrospinal fluid phospho-tau levels, a downstream marker of neuronal damage in AD, decreased with treatment among carriers receiving a lower dose of the medication (0.5 mg/

kg), while among noncarriers, they remained unchanged at 0.5 mg/kg but demonstrated a statistically significant decline in patients receiving a 1-mg/kg dose. The overall inference of these trials was that again there was a discrepancy between PET biomarker changes and clinical response. A pertinent concern raised with the use of amyloid PET agents has been that these techniques measure amyloid plaque burden, while neurotoxicity in AD is caused by fibrillary forms of β-amyloid in the preclinical course of the disease that are not imaged by the amyloid PET scans. Similarly, the lack of clinical efficacy of the antiamyloid antibody in these large trials has underscored the importance of exploring other biological therapeutic targets in AD in addition to β-amyloid, and newer PET tracers would be needed to facilitate those trials. Recently, a new class of radioligands targeting the 'tau' protein that leads to formation of intracellular neurofibrillary tangles in AD (e.g. [^{18}F]T807) has become available and further clinical studies are awaited [19].

Stroke

Internal carotid artery stenosis is a well-recognized etiology of transient ischemic attacks and strokes. Complete occlusion of the internal carotid artery is thought to cause 10–25% of ischemic stroke or transient ischemic attacks. The mechanism of stroke or transient ischemic attack in these patients may be related to hemodynamic consequences or due to an embolic phenomenon. The treatment of carotid artery occlusion has been controversial. Anticoagulation for variable intervals has been attempted. Surgical techniques to bypass the site of occlusion using an external carotid-internal carotid artery anastomosis (EC-IC bypass) have been used. An earlier randomized clinical trial performed in the mid-1980s showed no benefit of such a surgical procedure [20], but was criticized for not selecting patients with a hemodynamically significant stenosis who might have benefited more from the procedure as opposed to all patients. It was conjectured that a large proportion of the unselected population might have already developed significant hemodynamic compensation via collateral circulation. The Carotid Occlusion Surgery Study (COSS) was a subsequent multicenter randomized trial that selected patients with symptomatic internal carotid artery occlusion and increased oxygen extraction fraction (OEF) determined on $[^{15}O]H_2O$-PET and $[^{15}O]O_2$-PET, and randomized them to either EC-IC bypass plus medical therapy or medical therapy alone [21]. Mean regional carotid artery territory OEF was calculated using a 'quotient image' of $[^{15}O]O_2/[^{15}O]H_2O$ PET counts and an ipsilateral-to-contralateral ratio of OEF was calculated. A ratio cutoff of >1.130 was used to select patients for the trial [22]. A sample size of 394 was planned, but the trial was terminated early after recruiting 195 patients. At 2 years of follow-up in these patients, there was no difference in the primary end point between the surgical versus the nonsurgical arm (21 vs. 22.7%, p = 0.78). There was a significantly increased rate of ipsilateral stroke in the surgical arm in the first 30 days after the surgical procedure (14.3 vs. 2%). Numerous reasons have been cited for the failure of the trial including increased early postoperative morbidity in the surgical arm or unexpected effectiveness of medical therapy in the control arm.

Earlier Phase Trials

In addition to large phase III clinical trials, PET and SPECT imaging can be used to expedite and guide drug development in preclinical studies and earlier phases of clinical investigation [23]. This literature is substantial, but a detailed review of these studies is beyond the scope of this chapter.

Discussion

These examples illustrate both the advantages as well as challenges in using PET and SPECT for evidence-based research and clinical use in neurological disorders.

As noted above, in the clinical trials in both AD and Parkinson's disease, there was a mismatch between the findings on nuclear imaging and measured clinical outcomes. Thus, although PET and SPECT techniques could serve as biomarkers, they should not be considered 'surrogate end points' or a substitute for clinical end points. However, it needs to be emphasized that the changes seen using molecular imaging techniques may precede clinical changes by months or years, and longer follow-up may be needed to detect relevant clinical changes, which is not always feasible in large clinical trials. Similarly, there may be a mismatch between molecular imaging biomarkers and other nonimaging biomarkers as seen in some of the AD trials. These apparent discrepancies emphasize the need to further explore the underlying biological, methodological, and technical causes of the same. These insights would enable a better understanding of the underlying pathophysiology as well as improve methodological and technical approaches. In COSS [21], selection of patients based on an increased OEF did not alter the conclusions obtained from a previous trial [20] that attempted EC-IC bypass in unselected patients with internal carotid occlusion. In addition to the treatment-related reasons for the trial's failure already mentioned above, it is also possible that the selection of patients with 'hemodynamically significant' carotid artery occlusion was still not optimal in spite of randomizing only those patients who had an increased cerebral OEF. Increased OEF alone may not reflect the highest risk for stroke in patients with carotid occlusion, as demonstrated in a study by Derdeyn et al. [24] where patients with both increased OEF and cerebral blood volume (measured using $[^{15}O]$-labeled carbon monoxide) were shown to have much higher incidence of stroke than patients with increased OEF alone.

The lessons learned from these and other clinical trials emphasize that the considerations for successful use of PET or SPECT imaging as biomarkers in randomized trials for a neurological disease should include the following:

(1) In vivo behavior of the radiotracer and the imaging parameter studied should reflect a key aspect of the underlying pathology and/ or pathophysiology of the disease under question

(2) The underlying biological target and radiotracer distribution should have the potential to vary with treatment under study conditions, and adjustments must be made for any other known changes (e.g. physiological) that may occur over time

(3) Image reconstruction techniques and quantitative or semiquantitative image analysis approaches should be robust and standardized across trial sites

(4) Newer molecular targets should be explored based on insights obtained from basic science research and translational observations.

Hence, PET and SPECT have the potential to serve as invaluable biomarkers in randomized clinical trials of neurological disorders. Greater awareness and understanding about PET and SPECT among health professionals as well as the general public, along with a collaborative team including clinicians, imaging physicians, biologists, chemists, and physicists, among others, is needed for their successful implementation in clinical trials. These techniques have a highly significant potential to contribute to improving clinical outcomes and care for patients with neurological disorders.

References

1 Salter H, Holland R: Biomarkers: refining diagnosis and expediting drug development – reality, aspiration and the role of open innovation. J Intern Med 2014; 276:215–228.

2 Lesko LJ, Atkinson AJ Jr: Use of biomarkers and surrogate endpoints in drug development and regulatory decision making: criteria, validation, strategies. Ann Rev Pharmacol Toxicol 2001; 41:347 366.

3 James ML, Gambhir SS: A molecular imaging primer: modalities, imaging agents, and applications. Physiol Rev 2012;92:897–965.

4 Phelps ME: PET: a biological imaging technique. Neurochem Res 1991;16: 929–940.

5 Singhal T: Positron emission tomography applications in clinical neurology. Semin Neurol 2012;32:421–431.

6 Jones T, Rabiner EA; PET Research Advisory Company: The development, past achievements, and future directions of brain PET. J Cereb Blood Flow Metab 2012;32:1426–1454.

7 Fahn S, Oakes D, Shoulson I, et al: Levodopa and the progression of Parkinson's disease. N Engl J Med 2004;351: 2498–2508.

8 Djang DS, Janssen MJ, Bohnen N, et al: SNM practice guideline for dopamine transporter imaging with ^{123}I-ioflupane SPECT 1.0. J Nucl Med 2012;53:154–163.

9 Marek K, Seibyl J, Eberly S, et al: Longitudinal follow-up of SWEDD subjects in the PRECEPT study. Neurology 2014;80: 1791–1797.

10 Parkinson Study Group: Dopamine transporter brain imaging to assess the effects of pramipexole vs levodopa on Parkinson disease progression. JAMA 2002;287:1653–1661.

11 Asenbaum S, Brücke T, Pirker W, et al: Imaging of dopamine transporters with iodine-123-beta-CIT and SPECT in Parkinson's disease. J Nucl Med 1997;38: 1–6.

12 Seibyl JP, Marek KL, Quinlan D, et al: Decreased single-photon emission computed tomographic ^{123}I]beta-CIT striatal uptake correlates with symptom severity in Parkinson's disease. Ann Neurol 1995;38:589–598.

13 Marek K, Innis R, van Dyck C, et al: [123]I]beta-CIT SPECT imaging assessment of the rate of Parkinson's disease progression. Neurology 2001;57:2089–2894.

14 Morrish PK, Rakshi JS, Bailey DL, Sawle GV, Brooks DJ: Measuring the rate of progression and estimating the preclinical period of Parkinson's disease with [18F]dopa PET. J Neurol Neurosurg Psychiatry 1998;64:314–319.

15 Pavese N, Kiferle L, Piccini P: Neuroprotection and imaging studies in Parkinson's disease. Parkinsonism Relat Disord 2009;15(suppl 4):S33–S37.

16 Shah M, Seibyl J, Cartier A, Bhatt R, Catafau AM: Molecular imaging insights into neurodegeneration: focus on α-synuclein radiotracers. J Nucl Med 2014;55:1397–1400.

17 Rinne JO, Brooks DJ, Rossor MN, et al: ^{11}C-PiB PET assessment of change in fibrillar amyloid-beta load in patients with Alzheimer's disease treated with bapineuzumab: a phase 2, double-blind, placebo-controlled, ascending-dose study. Lancet Neurol 2010;9:363–372.

18 Salloway S, Sperling R, Fox NC, et al: Two phase 3 trials of bapineuzumab in mild-to-moderate Alzheimer's disease. N Engl J Med 2014;370:322–333.

19 Zimmer ER, Leuzy A, Gauthier S, Rosa-Neto P: Developments in tau PET imaging. Can J Neurol Sci 2014;41:547–553.

20 The EC/IC Bypass Study Group: Failure of extracranial-intracranial arterial bypass to reduce the risk of ischemic stroke. Results of an international randomized trial. N Engl J Med 1985;313: 1191–1200.

21 Powers WJ, Clarke WR, Grubb RL Jr, et al: Extracranial-intracranial bypass surgery for stroke prevention in hemodynamic cerebral ischemia: the Carotid Occlusion Surgery Study randomized trial. JAMA 2011;306:1983–1992.

22 Derdeyn CP, Videen TO, Simmons NR, et al: Count-based PET method for predicting ischemic stroke in patients with symptomatic carotid arterial occlusion. Radiology 1999;212:499–506.

23 Brooks DJ: Positron emission tomography and single-photon emission computed tomography in central nervous system drug development. NeuroRx 2005;2:226–236.

24 Derdeyn CP, Videen TO, Yundt KD, et al: Variability of cerebral blood volume and oxygen extraction: stages of cerebral haemodynamic impairment revisited. Brain 2002;125:595–607.

Tarun Singhal, MD
Department of Neurology, Brigham and Women's Hospital, Harvard Medical School
75 Francis Street
Boston, MA 02115 (USA)
E-Mail tsinghal@partners.org

Beghi E, Logroscino G (eds): The Right Therapy for Neurological Disorders. From Randomized Trials to Clinical Practice.
Front Neurol Neurosci. Basel, Karger, 2016, vol 39, pp 117–123 (DOI: 10.1159/000445452)

Cerebrospinal Fluid Biomarkers for Target Engagement and Efficacy in Clinical Trials for Alzheimer's and Parkinson's Diseases

Lucilla Parnetti[a] · Paolo Eusebi[a] · Alberto Lleó[b, c]

[a]Section of Neurology, Centre for Memory Disturbances, Ospedale S. Maria della Misericordia, Department of Medicine, University of Perugia, Perugia, Italy; [b]Memory Unit, Department of Neurology, Hospital de Sant Pau, Barcelona, and [c]Centro de Investigación Biomédica en Red en enfermedades Neurodegenerativas (CIBERNED), Madrid, Spain

Abstract

Background: Cerebrospinal fluid (CSF) is increasingly being used to detect biochemical changes that occur in different neurological conditions. In Alzheimer's disease (AD), three CSF biomarkers ($A\beta_{42}$, total tau, and phosphorylated tau) are used in clinical practice to support the diagnosis in the prodromal stages of the disease. In Parkinson's disease (PD), the investigation is following the pathway of AD research and some promising markers have been identified, with the main aim to favor an early diagnosis, i.e. in the premotor phase. Some of these CSF markers have also been incorporated in AD and PD clinical trials to demonstrate target engagement of the drug and/or to enrich the patient populations. In this chapter, we will review the main CSF biomarkers for AD and PD and their potential application to clinical trials. **Summary:** In clinical trials assessing the efficacy of disease-modifying agents for AD, CSF biomarkers are currently used both as a diagnostic criterion for inclusion and for monitoring the biochemical impact of the drug on the upstream neurodegenerative mechanisms. Accordingly, recent trials devoted to PD are following such a procedure, although in this neurodegenerative disorder CSF biomarkers are not ready yet for routine clinical use. **Key Messages:** AD and PD are neurodegenerative disorders that share a long asymptomatic/prodromal phase in which neurodegenerative phenomena already take place in the brain. Clinical trials assessing the efficacy of disease-modifying agents should include the CSF measurement of related biomarkers as biochemical proof of the underlying pathology as well as of the impact of the drug on these pathogenic mechanisms.

Alzheimer's disease (AD) and Parkinson's disease (PD) are the two most common neurodegenerative disorders. Current predictions estimate a progressive increase in the prevalence due to the age-related nature of both diseases and changes in population structure. Therefore, there is an urgent need to find therapeutic strategies to cure or slow the progression of AD and PD.

AD and PD both have a long preclinical and prodromal phase, in which brain changes occur with no or minimal symptoms. Characterizing these preclinical and prodromal phases is of critical importance for clinical practice and clinical trial design, as current studies indicate a lack of clinical improvement when interventions are carried out in the later stages of the disease. Over the last two decades, several biomarkers have been developed to track relevant pathophysiological processes that take place in the central nervous system in neurodegenerative diseases. The use of biomarkers is expected to facilitate an early and accurate diagnosis, and its application in clinical trials is expected to maximize the chances of success.

Cerebrospinal fluid (CSF) has been used for more than two decades as an accessible biological source to detect biochemical changes that occur in different neurological conditions. In AD, many CSF biomarkers have been investigated and some have reached clinical practice. In PD, the investigation is following the pathway of AD research and many promising markers have emerged. In this chapter, we will review the main CSF biomarkers for AD and PD and their potential application to clinical trials.

Cerebrospinal Fluid Biomarkers in Alzheimer's Disease and Parkinson's Disease

Alzheimer's Disease

Numerous studies have consistently identified a specific CSF biomarker signature that reflects the characteristic pathophysiological process of AD. AD patients typically show decreased levels of $A\beta_{42}$ (42-amino-acid-long amyloid-β) and increased levels of total tau (t-tau) and phosphorylated tau (p-tau) in CSF compared to cognitively normal individuals [1]. As these biomarkers reflect the neuropathological hallmarks of AD, these three biomarkers are often identified as *core* AD biomarkers. Core AD biomarkers have a sensitivity and specificity of over 80% in the diagnosis of AD dementia, and they are good prognostic markers to predict progression to dementia in patients with mild cognitive impairment [1]. Several studies using data obtained from the Alzheimer's disease Neuroimaging Initiative (ADNI) and other cohorts indicate that most patients with mild cognitive impairment with the typical AD signature progress to dementia within a 5-year period [1].

This biochemical signature has been incorporated in the National Institute on Aging – Alzheimer's Association (NIA-AA) criteria of AD [2, 3] and in the recently revised international research criteria for AD [4]. Under these criteria, the combination of the appropriate clinical syndrome (mild cognitive impairment or dementia) together with the biochemical AD signature can increase the level of certainty of the diagnosis of AD.

In addition to Aβ and tau, many other markers have been investigated to track further pathophysiological processes implicated in AD, or to detect common copathologies [5]. Markers of neuronal injury, inflammation, or synaptic loss are being investigated among others. These additional markers may not be specific of the pathophysiological process of AD, but may be useful prognostic or staging markers for clinical practice and in clinical trials.

Parkinson's Disease

Investigation of CSF as a potential source of biomarkers in PD [6] dates back to the 1960s. Reduced CSF monoamine concentrations (homovanillic acid and 5-hydroxyindoleacetic acid) were found in patients with parkinsonism and dementia [7].

Several studies have tested α-synuclein in human body fluids as a disease-linked candidate biomarker for PD. This was due to the observation that fibrillar aggregates called Lewy bodies in the substantia nigra are the histopathological hallmark of PD and α-synuclein is the main protein component of these aggregates [8]. Furthermore, the association between mutations in the α-synuclein gene (SNCA) and PD suggest a central role for α-synuclein in the disease process.

α-Synuclein is detectable in CSF [9–12], although quantification by ELISA and other similar assays have yielded heterogeneous results. The vast majority of the studies concluded that the deficit of α-synuclein clearance in the brain is followed by a reduction of total α-synuclein in CSF [11, 13, 14]. On the contrary, CSF oligomeric α-synuclein species are reported as increased in PD as well as in other synucleinopathies [14, 15].

Other biomarker candidates have been tested in recent years, and this area of research is growing rapidly. To this purpose, there has been high interest in recent years concerning lysosomal derangement in PD. GBA1 [the gene encoding for the lysosomal enzyme glucocerebrosidase (GCase)] mutations represent a recognized risk factor for PD and other parkinsonisms [16]; likewise, reduced activity of GCase has been reported both in the brain [17–19] and in CSF [14]. These findings are in agreement with the relationship existing between GCase activity and α-synuclein aggregation [20].

Classic AD biomarkers ($A\beta_{1-42}$, t-tau, and p-tau) have also been investigated in PD, mostly as prognostic biomarkers, with particular interest for detecting risk of cognitive decline in this condition.

A series of CSF biomarkers for oxidative stress, inflammation, and energy failure in parkinsonian disorders have also been investigated. Urate belongs to this set of biomarkers, being an endogenous antioxidant. Even though there is substantial evidence relating low serum levels of urate to PD, CSF studies have shown inconsistent results.

Cerebrospinal Fluid Biomarkers in Clinical Trials for Alzheimer's Disease

Many clinical trials for AD have incorporated CSF biomarkers as measures of target engagement and, less frequently, as a measure of disease progression or as a way to enrich the study with subjects with the typical pathophysiological process characteristic of AD. In this section, we will review the most used analytes and their potential usefulness in trials.

Aβ Peptides and Other Amyloid Precursor Protein Metabolites

$A\beta_{1-42}$ is the most investigated CSF biomarker in AD clinical trials (table 1). $A\beta_{1-42}$ levels have been systematically incorporated in many clinical trials of antiamyloid therapies as a measure of target engagement or for sample enrichment of patients in the early stages of AD. In trials with β-secretase or γ-secretase inhibitors, $A\beta_{1-42}$ levels in CSF have been mainly used to demonstrate target engagement of the drug. Most β-secretase inhibitors, such as LY2811376, LY2886721, E2609, or MK-8931, have markedly reduced Aβ levels in CSF in phase I–III trials, indicating strong enzymatic inhibition. Most trials with β-secretase inhibitors have also included the measurement of CSF levels of fragments derived from β-secretase cleavage of amyloid precursor protein (sAPPβ). CSF sAPPβ levels can reliably demonstrate drug target engagement and most trials with β-secretase inhibitors have shown up to 95% reductions [5].

Trials with γ-secretase inhibitors have also included $A\beta_{1-42}$ levels in CSF as proof of target engagement, and some trials have included the measurement of $A\beta_{1-15}$ and/or $A\beta_{1-16}$ levels, as they increase in response to γ-secretase inhibition. Although trials of γ-secretase in AD have been discontinued due to adverse effects, the use of CSF biomarkers has clearly aided clinical development by showing target engagement.

Trials with active or passive antiamyloid immunization have also included $A\beta_{1-42}$ levels in CSF. Active immunization with AN1792 or CAD-106, or passive immunization with bapineuzumab showed no effect on CSF $A\beta_{1-42}$ levels. However, treatment with the antiamyloid antibody solanezumab increased total $A\beta_{1-42}$ and $A\beta_{1-40}$ levels in CSF, suggesting mobilization of the central Aβ pool. The differential effects of bapineuzumab and solanezumab on CSF $A\beta_{1-42}$ are believed to be due to the fact that solanezumab was designed to target soluble Aβ while bapineuzumab mainly targets fibrillar Aβ. In a phase II study of the γ-secretase inhibitor avagacestat, CSF $A\beta_{1-42}$ levels (or high tau/$A\beta_{1-42}$ ratio) were used to select patients with prodromal AD. Unfortunately, the clinical development of avagacestat was terminated due to insufficient target engagement. CSF $A\beta_{1-42}$ levels were also used in the

Table 1. Clinical trials of the main strategies in AD and PD that used CSF biomarkers

Drug	Population	Phase	Biomarker use	Outcome
Alzheimer's disease β-Secretase inhibitors	Healthy volunteers to AD dementia	I–III	Target engagement	↓A$β_{1-42}$; ↑A$β_{5-40}$; ↓sAPPβ
γ-Secretase inhibitors	Healthy volunteers to AD dementia	I–III	Target engagement Enrichment	↓A$β_{1-42}$; ↑A$β_{1-14/16}$
Active Aβ immunotherapy	Healthy volunteers to AD dementia	I–II	Disease modification	= A$β_{1-42}$ ↓tau
Passive Aβ immunotherapy	Healthy volunteers to AD dementia	I–III	Target engagement Disease modification Enrichment	= A$β_{1-42}$ ↑A$β_{1-40}$ ↑A$β_{1-42}$ (solanezumab) ↓p-tau (bapineuzumab)
Parkinson's disease Selegiline and tocopherol	PD	III	Disease modification Target engagement	= Homovanillic acid (tocopherol) ↓ Homovanillic acid (selegiline)
PD01A	PD	I	Disease modification Target engagement	NA
sNN0031	PD	I	Target engagement	NA
Inosine	PD	II	Target engagement	↑ Urate
Deferiprone	PD	II	Target engagement	↓ Ferritin and oxidative markers

For further references see Lleó et al. [5].

phase III trial of the antiamyloid antibody gantenerumab to select patients with prodromal or mild AD, but no data have been released yet.

Finally, CSF A$β_{1-42}$ levels have also been determined as exploratory analysis in some trials of non-amyloid-based therapies, usually as an indicator of disease modification.

In summary, the available data on AD indicate that CSF Aβ levels can reliably be used as a measure of target engagement in trials with β-secretase and γ-secretase inhibitors, although the interpretation in the case of immunization trials poses more challenges.

Tau and Phosphorylated Tau

T-tau and p-tau levels in CSF have been used in many clinical trials with amyloid or non-amyloid-based therapies as indicators or disease modification. Trials with β- or γ-secretase inhibitors have failed to detect differences in t-tau or p-tau levels. However, active or passive Aβ immunization strategies have shown changes in t-tau or p-tau levels, although the interpretation is not always straightforward. Data from the active Aβ immunization trials with AN1792 have indicated that treatment reduced t-tau levels in CSF. This finding may indicate an effect of the drug on the intensity of neuronal degeneration due to direct or indirect effects of cortical Aβ removal. Data from phase II and III trials with bapineuzumab indicate that treatment reduced p-tau levels in CSF. This finding suggests that bapineuzumab may reduce tau phosphorylation in the brain, although this change was not associated with any clinical benefit. In contrast, treatment with the monoclonal Aβ solanezumab did not change tau levels in the phase III trials. The fact that solanezumab was designed to bind soluble Aβ and that bapineuzumab and AN1792 also target fibrillar Aβ suggest that changes in fibrillar Aβ are more connected with markers of neurodegeneration than are changes in soluble Aβ. Many other clinical trials with amyloid- and non-amyloid-based strategies have incorporated t-tau and p-tau as measures of disease modification or for exploratory analysis (table 1).

Tau-Independent Markers of Neuronal Injury
A number of tau-independent markers of neuronal damage are being investigated in AD, such as neurofilaments, heart fatty acid-binding protein, and visinin-like protein 1. These markers may be particularly useful in trials with anti-tau strategies as additional measures of disease modification, as tau levels under these conditions may reflect target engagement instead of neuronal damage.

Synaptic markers, such as neurogranin or SNAP-25, have also been investigated in AD. The positive correlation observed for these markers with disease progression makes them good candidates for future clinical trials.

Neuroinflammation Markers
Markers of CSF microglial activation such as chitotriosidase, chitinase-3-like protein 1 (also known as YKL-40), and C-C motif chemokine 2 may be additional useful markers for clinical trials of AD. The levels of these markers are elevated in early AD and may correlate with disease progression [5, 21]. Although markers of neuroinflammation are not specific to AD, they may serve to monitor disease progression in clinical trials.

Others
Comorbidities are common in patients with neurodegenerative diseases in general and with AD in particular. The presence of comorbidities may have important implications for clinical trials since these coincident pathologies may not be targeted by a specific drug. Markers to detect these common comorbidities are an important area of research. α-Synuclein in CSF has been investigated as a potential marker of Lewy body pathology and TAR DNA-binding protein 43 in CSF has been explored to detect TAR DNA-binding protein 43 pathology.

Cerebrospinal Fluid Biomarkers in Clinical Trials for Parkinson's Disease

The underuse of CSF biomarkers in PD, both in observational and randomized studies, is due to the absence of valid candidates. However, a few clinical trials have analyzed CSF as a source of efficacy and/or target engagement, or for exploratory purposes (table 1).

Dopamine Metabolites
CSF levels of dopamine and its metabolites have been used as measures of PD progression in clinical trials. Levels of homovanillic acid in CSF were included as a secondary outcome measure in the DATATOP trial, which evaluated the efficacy of selegiline and tocopherol in patients with PD. CSF concentrations of homovanillic acid were reduced in patients treated with selegiline, indicating positive target engagement [22].

α-Synuclein
CSF α-synuclein is now being explored as a surrogate marker of efficacy and/or target engagement in patients with PD or other synucleinopathies. Active immunization with α-synuclein in patients with PD is being investigated in a phase I study with the PD01A peptide-carrier conjugate vaccine (table 1). The study will include titration of PD01A-induced antibodies and α-synuclein CSF levels.

Others
A phase II trial of inosine, an orally bioavailable central nervous system-penetrant purine precursor of urate, is also under scrutiny in patients with

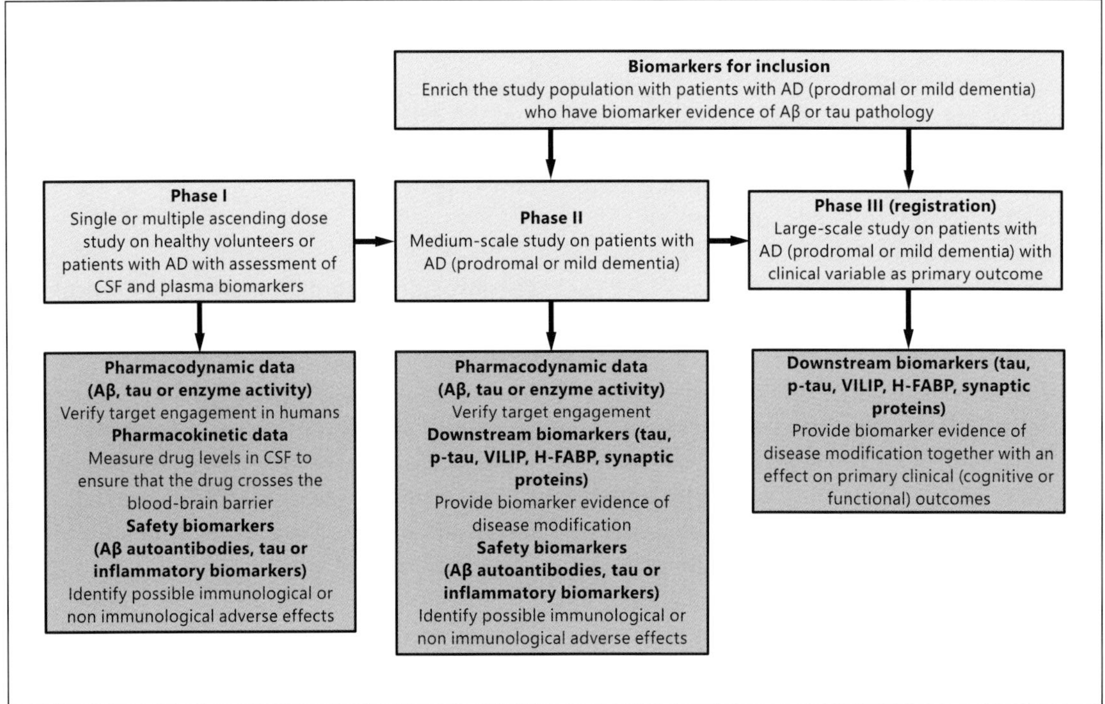

Fig. 1. Position of CSF biomarkers in AD clinical trials. Flowchart to illustrate how CSF biomarkers can be implemented in the different phases of clinical trials with disease-modifying agents for patients with AD. This scheme assumes that the drug candidate has been found to have an acceptable pharmacokinetic profile in preclinical development, and that studies in AD transgenic models have indicated an effect on amyloid and/or tau pathology. H-FABP = Heart fatty acid-binding protein; VILIP = visinin-like protein 1. With permission from Lleó et al. [5].

PD. Serial CSF samples are being taken to evaluate urate levels in CSF.

A phase II study tested the effect of the iron chelator deferiprone in patients with PD. The results indicated that treatment with deferiprone reduced brain iron overload as detected by MRI, as well as levels of ferritin and markers of oxidative stress in CSF [23].

sNN0031, a recombinant human platelet-derived growth factor (rhPDGF), is being tested in a phase I study in patients with PD. Intracerebroventricular administration of recombinant human PDGF had a positive effect on dopaminergic denervation, and serial CSF samples were taken to measure PDGF levels aiming at monitoring target engagement [24].

Conclusions

Current CSF biomarkers are useful in AD clinical trials for enriching patient samples and for demonstrating positive target engagement (fig. 1). However, the relationship between the effects of a drug on one or more CSF biomarkers and some clinical outcomes is often uncertain. A recent phase III trial of amyloid-lowering agents in AD showed that the biomarker levels and clinical responses were not related.

In PD research, the biomarker field is moving forward and current trials are incorporating CSF biomarkers mainly to measure target engagement.

Standardization of preanalytical and analytical variables, including the development of fully automated assays and the definition of global cutoffs, is still a major concern in CSF biomarkers for PD. Novel biomarkers are needed in PD but also in AD, especially markers with a strong link with disease modification (e.g. synaptic pro-teins). The use of CSF biomarkers in clinical trials can guide clinical development by ensuring target engagement and downstream effects of the drug.

References

1 Blennow K, Hampel H, Weiner M, Zetterberg H: Cerebrospinal fluid and plasma biomarkers in Alzheimer disease. Nat Rev Neurol 2010;6:131–144.

2 McKhann GM, Knopman DS, Chertkow H, et al: The diagnosis of dementia due to Alzheimer's disease: recommendations from the National Institute on Aging-Alzheimer's Association workgroups on diagnostic guidelines for Alzheimer's disease. Alzheimers Dement 2011;7:263–269.

3 Albert MS, DeKosky ST, Dickson D, et al: The diagnosis of mild cognitive impairment due to Alzheimer's disease: recommendations from the National Institute on Aging-Alzheimer's Association workgroups on diagnostic guidelines for Alzheimer's disease. Alzheimers Dement 2011;7:270–279.

4 Dubois B, Feldman HH, Jacova C, et al: Advancing research diagnostic criteria for Alzheimer's disease: the IWG-2 criteria. Lancet Neurol 2014;13:614–629.

5 Lleó A, Cavedo E, Parnetti L, et al: Cerebrospinal fluid biomarkers for Alzheimer's and Parkinson's disease and their application in clinical trials. Nat Rev Neurol 2015;11:41–55.

6 Magdalinou N, Lees AJ, Zetterberg H: Cerebrospinal fluid biomarkers in parkinsonian conditions: an update and future directions. J Neurol Neurosurg Psychiatry 2014;85:1065–1075.

7 Gottfries CG, Gottfries I, Roos BE: Homovanillic acid and 5-hydroxyindoleacetic acid in the cerebrospinal fluid of patients with senile dementia, presenile dementia and parkinsonism. J Neurochem 1969;16:1341–1345.

8 Spillantini MG, Schmidt ML, Lee VM, Trojanowski JQ, Jakes R, Goedert M: α-Synuclein in Lewy bodies. Nature 1997;388:839–840.

9 Borghi R, Marchese R, Negro A, et al: Full length alpha-synuclein is present in cerebrospinal fluid from Parkinson's disease and normal subjects. Neurosci Lett 2000;253:13–16.

10 El-Agnaf OM, Salem SA, Paleologou KE, et al: Alpha-synuclein implicated in Parkinson's disease is present in extracellular biological fluids, including human plasma. FASEB J 2003;17:1945–1947.

11 Tokuda T, Salem SA, Allsop D, et al: Decreased α-synuclein in cerebrospinal fluid of aged individuals and subjects with Parkinson's disease. Biochem Biophys Res Commun 2006;349:162–166.

12 Mollenhauer B, Cullen V, Kahn I, et al: Direct quantification of CSF α-synuclein by ELISA and first cross- sectional study in patients with neurodegeneration. Exp Neurol 2008;213:315–325.

13 Hong Z, Shi M, Chung KA, et al: DJ-1 and alpha-synuclein in human cerebrospinal fluid as biomarkers of Parkinson's disease. Brain 2010;133:713–726.

14 Parnetti L, Chiasserini D, Persichetti E, et al: Cerebrospinal fluid lysosomal enzymes and alpha-synuclein in Parkinson's disease. Mov Disord 2014;29:1019–1027.

15 Tokuda T, Qureshi MM, Ardah MT, et al: Detection of elevated levels of α-synuclein oligomers in CSF from patients with Parkinson disease. Neurology 2010;75:1766–1772.

16 Sidransky E, Nalls MA, Aasly JO, et al: Multicenter analysis of glucocerebrosidase mutations in Parkinson's disease. N Engl J Med 2009;361:1651–1661.

17 Gegg ME, Burke D, Heales SJ, et al: Glucocerebrosidase deficiency in substantia nigra of Parkinson disease brains. Ann Neurol 2012;72:455–463.

18 Murphy KE, Gysbers AM, Abbott SK, et al: Reduced glucocerebrosidase is associated with increased α-synuclein in sporadic Parkinson's disease. Brain 2014;137:834–848.

19 Chiasserini D, Paciotti S, Eusebi P, et al: Selective loss of glucocerebrosidase activity in sporadic Parkinson's disease and dementia with Lewy bodies. Mol Neurodegener 2015;10:15.

20 Mazzulli JR, Xu YH, Sun Y, et al: Gaucher disease glucocerebrosidase and α-synuclein form a bidirectional pathogenic loop in synucleinopathies. Cell 2011;146:37–52.

21 Alcolea D, Carmona-Iragui M, Suárez-Calvet M, et al: Relationship between β-secretase, inflammation and core cerebrospinal fluid biomarkers for Alzheimer's disease. J Alzheimers Dis 2014;42:157–167.

22 DATATOP: a multicenter controlled clinical trial in early Parkinson's disease. Parkinson Study Group. Arch Neurol 1989;46:1052–1060.

23 Devos D, Moreau C, Devedjian JC, et al: Targeting chelatable iron as a therapeutic modality in Parkinson's disease. Antioxid Redox Signal 2014;21:195–201.

24 Paul-Visse G, Zachrisson O, Varrone A, et al: Safety and efficacy of recombinant human platelet derived growth factor BB (rhPDGF-BB) in Parkinson's disease (abstract 487). Mov Disord 2013;28(suppl 1):S173.

Lucilla Parnetti
Clinica Neurologica, Centro Disturbi della Memoria
Ospedale S. Maria della Misericordia
S. Andrea delle Fratte
IT–06132 Perugia (Italy)
E-Mail lucilla.parnetti@unipg.it

Beghi E, Logroscino G (eds): The Right Therapy for Neurological Disorders. From Randomized Trials to Clinical Practice.
Front Neurol Neurosci. Basel, Karger, 2016, vol 39, pp 124–135 (DOI: 10.1159/000445453)

Pharmacogenetics in Neurodegenerative Diseases: Implications for Clinical Trials

Rosanna Tortelli[a, b] · Davide Seripa[c] · Francesco Panza[a–c] · Vincenzo Solfrizzi[d] · Giancarlo Logroscino[a, b]

[a]Neurodegenerative Disease Unit, Department of Basic Medicine, Neuroscience and Sense Organs, University of Bari 'Aldo Moro', Bari, [b]Department of Clinical Research in Neurology, University of Bari 'Aldo Moro', 'Pia Fondazione Cardinale G. Panico', Tricase, [c]Geriatric Unit and Laboratory of Gerontology and Geriatrics, Department of Medical Sciences, IRCCS 'Casa Sollievo della Sofferenza', San Giovanni Rotondo, and [d]Geriatric Medicine-Memory Unit and Rare Disease Centre, University of Bari 'Aldo Moro', Bari, Italy

Abstract

Background: Pharmacogenetics has become extremely important over the last 20 years for identifying individuals more likely to be responsive to pharmacological interventions. The role of genetic background as a predictor of drug response is a young and mostly unexplored field in neurodegenerative diseases. ***Summary:*** Mendelian mutations in neurodegenerative diseases have been used as models for early diagnosis and intervention. On the other hand, genetic polymorphisms or risk factors for late-onset Alzheimer's disease (AD) or other neurodegenerative diseases, probably influencing drug response, are hardly taken into account in randomized clinical trial (RCT) design. The same is true for genetic variants in cytochrome P450 (CYP), the principal enzymes influencing drug metabolism. A better characterization of individual genetic background may optimize clinical trial design and personal drug response. This chapter describes the state of the art about the impact of genetic factors in RCTs on neurodegenerative disease, with AD, frontotemporal dementia, Parkinson's disease, amyotrophic lateral scle- rosis, and Huntington's disease as examples. Furthermore, a brief description of the genetic bases of drug response focusing on neurodegenerative diseases will be conducted. ***Key Messages:*** The role of pharmacogenetics in RCTs for neurodegenerative diseases is still a young, unexplored, and promising field. Genetic tools allow increased sophistication in patient profiling and treatment optimization. Pharmaceutical companies are aware of the value of collecting genetic data during their RCTs. Pharmacogenetic research is bidirectional with RCTs: efficacy data are correlated with genetic polymorphisms, which in turn define subjects for treatment stratification.

© 2016 S. Karger AG, Basel

Pharmacogenetics is the science and clinical application of genetics to pharmacological treatments, i.e. determining if interindividual differences in drug efficacy and toxicity are due to genetic differences, identifying the genes that influence drug response, and using the genotype to predict outcome, and thus maximizing benefits and averting side effects.

Over the last 40 years, genetics has made a huge contribution in the understanding of pathological mechanisms involved in neurodegeneration. The best example is represented by the monogenic forms of early-onset (<65 years) Alzheimer's disease (AD), related to mutations in amyloid precursor protein, presenilin (PSEN)-1, and PSEN-2. The discovery of these three genes corroborated the involvement of the β-amyloid (Aβ) peptide as central to AD pathogenesis, addressing possible Aβ-based AD therapeutics with disease-modifying potential and priming the era of randomized clinical trials (RCTs) of immunotherapy in AD [1]. However, all the RCTs on immunotherapy in AD have failed to produce positive results to date or have been interrupted due to severe side effects. On the other hand, the only recognized risk factor and phenotypic modifier for late-onset AD is apolipoprotein E (APOE), which is also the most studied polymorphism in humans, associated with neurodegenerative and autoimmune diseases [2, 3]. Genetics is also important for other neurodegenerative diseases, such as the frontotemporal dementia (FTD)/amyotrophic lateral sclerosis (ALS) spectrum, mostly linked to mutations in progranulin (GRN), microtubule-associated protein tau, superoxide dismutase 1 (SOD1), TAR DNA-binding protein, fused in sarcoma/translocate in liposarcoma, and chromosome 9 open reading frame 72 (C9orf72) genes [4, 5], as well as the Parkinson's disease (PD) spectrum with mutations in the series of 18 specific chromosomal regions, also called chromosomal loci, termed PARK (to denote their putative link to PD), and numbered in chronological order of their identification (PARK1 to PARK18) [6]. In the majority of cases, genetically determined neurodegenerative diseases are phenotypically indistinguishable from nongenetic forms, even though many specific genotype-phenotype correlations have been described. It is clear that the clinical phenotypes resulting from mutations in these genes, and also from mutations in the same gene, may be different and thus respond differently to drugs/treatments. These are variables that must be taken into account when designing an RCT.

The genetic factors potentially influencing RCTs in neurodegenerative diseases may be identified as part of three clusters: (1) genetic factors causing a disease, (2) genetic factors associated with, but not the cause of, a disease, and (3) genetic factors affecting drug metabolism. This classification automatically arranges neurodegenerative diseases across the first two clusters in which the autosomal dominant/recessive inherited forms (early onset) are in the first and the sporadic forms (more resembling to complex disease) are in the second ones, virtually unhooking the third cluster but linking it with drug metabolism. It must be noted that the first cluster of genetic factors is not independent from the second one. Thus, those patients carrying a genetic factor causing neurodegenerative diseases (e.g. a PSEN-1 mutation) may be also carriers of a genetic factor associated with, but not the cause of, the disease that may influence the clinical phenotype. This should be taken into account in the design of any RCT on neurodegenerative diseases; however, it is almost never done in the real world. This chapter is going to describe the impact of genetic factors in RCTs on neurodegenerative disease, with AD, FTD, PD, ALS, and Huntington's disease (HD) as examples. Furthermore, a brief description of the genetic bases of drug response, focusing on neurodegenerative diseases, will be conducted.

Impact of Genetic Factors in Randomized Clinical Trials on Alzheimer's Disease

Referring to genetic factors causing disease, the monogenic forms of AD have been taken into account as ideal models for preventive RCTs. Among prevention/early treatment trials, it is important to mention the Dominantly Inherited Alzheimer Network (DIAN) [7] started in 2012 to analyze subjects who are carriers of autosomal dominant genetic mutations, and therefore at very high risk to develop AD at an early age. DIAN is testing two different anti-Aβ monoclonal antibodies: solanezumab and gantenerumab (table 1). In the DIAN trial, primary outcome measures are the amount of fibrillar amyloid deposition as measured by ^{11}C-labeled Pittsburgh compound B positron emission tomography scans for gantenerumab, while for solanezumab they are the concentrations of cerebrospinal fluid Aβ species at baseline and at the 2-year follow-up. This trial aims to enroll 210 individuals and the principal inclusion criteria are 18–80 years of age, individuals who know they have an AD-causing mutation or are unaware of their genetic status and have a 50% chance of having an autosomal dominant AD mutation (e.g. parent or sibling with a known AD-causing mutation), and individuals who are within –15 to +10 years of their parental age of symptom onset and cognitively normal or with mild cognitive impairment or mild dementia, Clinical Dementia Rating Scale of 0–1 (inclusive) [8].

Finally, a secondary prevention trial with the anti-Aβ monoclonal antibody crenezumab started in 2013, the Alzheimer's Prevention Initiative (API), is recruiting 300 individuals who are 30 years of age or older and symptom free, from the world's largest early-onset AD kindred in Antioquia, Colombia, with a mutant gene (PSEN-1 E280A) associated with a dominant form of early-onset AD (table 1). The PSEN-1 E280A mutation leads to early and robust cerebral $A\beta_{1-42}$ plaque deposition at a relatively young age [9], which is followed within 10–15 years, around age 50, by a progressive decline in cognition and clinical function, which is decades before the typical sporadic AD cases [10]. This extraordinary kindred, which has been followed for more than 20 years, includes about 5,000 people, with a sufficient number of presymptomatic carriers in the targeted age

group to make it possible to relate a treatment's effects on both biomarker and clinical end points within 2–5 years [11]. In the API trial, which has a 5-year treatment period, 100 PSEN-1 mutation carriers are receiving monthly injections of crenezumab, 100 are getting placebo, and 100 noncarriers are receiving placebo – the study participants are not told whether they carry the pathogenic mutation or not [8].

In these RCTs, the genetic background is a fundamental aid in discovering new preventive therapies. Genetic background is also important if we consider genetic factors associated with, but not the cause of, disease. As mentioned before, APOE is the strongest phenotypic modifier in late-onset AD. It is also the only genetic marker able to influence drug response and taken into account in RCTs on AD. Association of APOE ε4 with increased risk and earlier age at onset (AAO) of late-onset AD was first reported in 1993 [12, 13]. Twenty years ago, for the first time, the effects of APOE genotype on clinical response to treatment with tacrine, the first acetylcholinesterase inhibitor (AchEI) approved by the US Food and Drug Administration (FDA) for the management of AD symptoms, were examined [14]. The findings from AD autopsy studies suggesting that APOE ε4 presence is associated with decreased numbers of cholinergic markers in the temporal cortex and the hippocampus gave rise to the hypothesis that cholinergic therapy might have been less effective in APOE ε4 carriers. This hypothesis was confirmed by the findings of this study, suggesting that the APOE genotype may be a predictor of clinical response to tacrine in AD patients, with the APOE ε4 carriers associated with a lower probability of cognitive improvement [14]. However, these findings were not confirmed for other AchEIs, such as metrifonate, rivastigmine, and galantamine [15–17].

Genetic background was not taken into consideration in clinical trials on sporadic AD until the RCT with rosiglitazone, an agonist of the peroxisome proliferator-activated receptor that

Table 1. Principal secondary prevention trials of monoclonal antibodies targeting Aβ for the treatment of AD

Trial Compound (Company) Collaborators Clinical Trials.gov Identifier	Binding characteristics	Estimated or completed enrollment	Characteristics	Status
Antiamyloid treatment in asymptomatic AD (A4)				
Solanezumab (Eli Lilly) (LY2062430)	Humanized monoclonal IgG1 anti-Aβ$_{1-42}$ antibody (Aβ$_{13-28}$), binding-soluble Aβ			
NCT02008357		1,000 patients (2014–2018)	400 mg administered once every 4 weeks by intravenous infusion for 168 weeks	Phase III trial (currently recruiting)
Dominantly Inherited Alzheimer Network-Trials Unit (DIAN-TU)				
Solanezumab (Eli Lilly) (LY2062430)	Humanized monoclonal IgG1 anti-Aβ$_{1-42}$ antibody (Aβ$_{13-28}$), binding-soluble Aβ			
Gantenerumab (Hoffmann-La Roche) (RO4909832) Washington University School of Medicine Alzheimer's Association National Institute on Aging (NIA) Avid Radiopharmaceuticals	Fully human monoclonal IgG1 antibody against Aβ$_{1-42}$ (Aβ$_{1-10}$ and Aβ$_{19-26}$), not binding-soluble Aβ			
NCT01760005		210 patients (2012–2017)	Solanezumab: 400 mg intravenous infusion every 4 weeks for 2 years Gantenerumab: 225 mg subcutaneously every 4 weeks for 2 years	Phase II/III trial (currently recruiting)
Alzheimer's Prevention Initiative (API)				
Crenezumab (Genentech) (MABT5102A); Banner Alzheimer's Institute	Humanized monoclonal IgG4 antibody against Aβ$_{1-42}$ (Aβ$_{12-23}$)			
NCT01998841		300 patients (2013–2020)	Crenezumab subcutaneous injections every 2 weeks for 260 weeks	Phase II trial (currently recruiting)

increases glucose sensitivity, regulates lipid metabolism, and promotes mitochondrial biogenesis in mild-to-moderate AD patients. In 2006, a phase II RCT of rosiglitazone in mild-to-moderate AD patients showed, in a post hoc analysis, a clear improvement in cognitive performances for the highest dose only in APOE ε4 noncarriers [18]. Therefore, genotype-related efficacy was proposed, and an APOE-specific design was adopted for the phase III RCT, using a priori stratification of patients according to genotype (APOE ε4-negative and APOE ε4-positive patients) [19]. Unfortunately, this phase III RCT did not show any evidence of efficacy [19].

More recently, a phase II RCT with bapineuzumab, the first passive anti-Aβ immunotherapy with monoclonal antibodies for AD, was characterized by a higher frequency of vasogenic edema in APOE ε4 carriers, but failed to reach the primary outcome, except for slight differences in some clinical measures in APOE ε4 noncarriers identified in post hoc analysis [20]. These findings highlighted the role of genotype for RCTs in AD and led to the inclusion of the APOE genotype in the study design of the two subsequent phase III RCTs, one involving 1,121 carriers of APOE ε4 and the other 1,331 noncarriers [21]. There were no differences in drug response, but the authors found differences in AD-related biomarkers only in APOE ε4 carriers [21]. In particular, bapineuzumab-treated patients had reduced cerebrospinal fluid phospho-tau concentrations and, among APOE ε4 carriers, a decreased rate of accumulation of cortical amyloid in the brain on ^{11}C-labeled Pittsburgh compound B positron emission tomography [21]. It was therefore clear that a different genotype could be very important in drug response and in side-effect occurrence also in neurodegenerative diseases.

Despite the high importance of genotype in drug response, subsequent phase III RCTs on AD or other neurodegenerative disorders hardly considered genotype in their design, or even in the post hoc analysis. This is probably due to a still 'fuzzy' scenario in which it is often not clear which genes have been shown to be a determinant in the response to a specific drug in a specific disease.

The importance of genetic background in RCT design for AD has been reproposed in the past 2 years. In dementias, but also in other neurodegenerative diseases, the AAO is the most relevant prognostic determinant. Delaying the AAO of AD a few years would have a great impact on the global health of the aging world. Modelling studies have suggested that up to 40% of variability in the AAO of AD may be heritable, but is largely unknown. The APOE genotype only explains about 10% of variation, with a reduction of up to 7–9 years for each ε4 allele [22]. In 2007, fine mapping of the region within and surrounding APOE identified a new gene of interest, TOMM40, in linkage disequilibrium with the APOE ε4 allele [23]. Sequencing identified a variable length poly-T repeat sequence in intron 6 of TOMM40 that contributed to influence the AAO of AD, in the sense that individuals with APOE ε3/ε4 genotype and long poly-T repeats (defined as ≥27) had significantly lower AAO of AD than individuals with APOE ε3/ε4 genotype and short repeats [24]. The identification of TOMM40 as a strong modifier of disease triggered many efforts to test drugs that could delay the AAO using a biomarker risk algorithm. In fact, the only other example of a genotype-based RCT design for AD is the TOMMORROW trial, an ongoing large phase III RCT that is evaluating the role of pioglitazone, a drug that increases the number of mitochondria, in delaying the onset of the disease depending on genetic biomarkers (APOE/TOMM40) [25]. This RCT is testing a low dose of pioglitazone to determine whether it may delay the onset of mild cognitive impairment due to AD in cognitively normal subjects at high risk of developing disease within the period of the trial [26]. This is the first example of a trial using a genetic prognostic trait to stratify patients, beyond APOE status.

Impact of Genetic Factors in Randomized Clinical Trials on Frontotemporal Dementia and Amyotrophic Lateral Sclerosis

FTD is a neurodegenerative disorder usually presenting with either behavioral or language impairment, although it has significant overlap with motor neuron disease and the atypical parkinsonian disorders [27, 28]. The clinical evidence of overlap between FTD and motor neuron disease has recently gained support after the C9orf72 mutation was found to be the most common genetic abnormality in familial and sporadic forms of both FTD and ALS, particularly frequent in patients and families with both conditions [29, 30]. At present, there are no treatments that can delay the onset or prevent the progression of genetic FTD. Evidence from other neurodegenerative diseases, as seen above for AD, shows that there are changes in a number of biomarkers many years before symptom onset, suggesting that the ideal time for treating these disorders is likely to be prior to clinical presentation. The identification of robust biomarkers in genetic FTD that are indicative of disease onset and progression are therefore prerequisites for any disease-modifying treatment. Ideally, therapies should have been instituted when the minimum of irreversible neuronal loss has occurred, making RCT design challenging and increasing the importance of biomarkers in selecting suitable subjects and in monitoring progression.

Unfortunately, there are still no biomarkers of genetic FTD that can confidently predict when a disease-modifying treatment should be initiated or how the response to it should be monitored. The only robust and clinically accepted biomarker is decreased plasma levels of progranulin in GRN mutation carriers. Decreased plasma progranulin concentrations are found in symptomatic patients with GRN mutations, but similarly low levels have also been found in presymptomatic mutation carriers who are in their 20s and 30s, and therefore many years prior to disease onset [31, 32]. For GRN mutations, a uniform disease mechanism of loss of progranulin function operates in all mutation carriers, and drugs such as chloroquine, nimodipine, and vorinostat have been shown to increase progranulin concentration [33, 34], suggesting their possible use in future preventive RCTs. Based upon these models, the Genetic Frontotemporal Dementia Initiative (GENFI) was set up in 2011 to bring together research centers across Europe and Canada with an interest in clinical studies of presymptomatic genetic FTD.

In ALS, there are only a few RCTs that have adopted a priori or a posteriori stratification of patients according to the presence of mutations in one of the known genes, even though they often influence the phenotype. This is understandable for SOD1, TAR DNA-binding protein, fused in sarcoma, or other genes with low frequency, especially in sporadic cases. It is less understandable for C9orf72 G_4C_2 expansion, which has a frequency of up to 50% in familial cases and up to 10% in sporadic ones, and which strongly influences phenotype in terms of prognosis directly or through the association with frontotemporal cognitive decline [35]. Before one can translate these findings into new causal or modifying therapies, better insights into the exact pathogenic mechanisms are essential, which should result in the development of a completely new class of therapeutic strategies. However, emerging technologies in antisense oligonucleotides and RNA silencing are promising as novel therapeutic strategies targeting specific genes in familial ALS, such as SOD1 and C9orf72 [36]. Their therapeutic potential was recently demonstrated by the phase I trial of the intrathecal delivery of antisense oligonucleotide ISIS 333611 in SOD1 patients with familial ALS [37]. A major problem in translating preclinical findings into new treatments for ALS patients is the lack of reproducibility of the preclinical studies. Recently, the ALS Therapy Development Institute (TDI) retested different compounds with a reported beneficial effect in the mutant SOD1 mouse model. Unfortunately, TDI was unable to obtain any beneficial effect in humans [38].

Impact of Genetic Factors in Randomized Clinical Trials on Parkinson's Disease and Huntington's Disease

Most pharmacological approaches to the treatment of PD are symptomatic and target the nigrostriatal dopaminergic pathway [39]. Loss of dopamine, once considered the cause of PD, is now questioned as the initial event in PD pathogenesis and is certainly not the only viable pathway. Responses to L-DOPA and other dopamine agonists, as well as side effects, consistently vary among individuals, and this is largely determined by genetic background. The pharmacogenetics of PD consists of association studies with genes whose products directly interact with L-DOPA, dopamine, or dopamine agonists, i.e. COMT, MAO-A, MAO-B, dopamine transporter (DAT), and dopamine receptors (DRD1, DRD2, DRD3, DRD4, and DRD5) [39]. It is nearly impossible to determine whether and which dopamine-related polymorphisms are important for dose determination, avoiding side effects, or predicting a positive response. There are several reasons for this, which include disparity in study designs, small sample sizes, and lack of replication. Furthermore, at present, no genome-wide association study has been designed specifically to assess response to PD drugs or for prevention of the disease. However, two genome-wide gene-drug interaction studies showed that the caffeine effect on PD risk reduction was associated with polymorphisms in GRIN2A, which encodes the NMDA glutamate receptor subunit 2A [40], and that the nicotine effect was associated with polymorphisms in SV2C encoding the synaptic vesicle protein 2C [41]. GRIN2A and SV2C may also be useful for stratifying patients in RCTs on PD.

Finally, HD is a progressive and fatal neurodegenerative disease caused by CAG repeat expansions in the gene encoding huntingtin. This is the best example of a disease-causing gene that can be targeted in RCTs. However, every attempt to prevent or slow its progression in patients and muta-tion carriers has failed so far [42]. The known genetic cause of HD allows targeting the known pathogenic entity, mutant huntingtin protein (mHTT). Lowering the expression of mHTT at the level of DNA (transcription) or RNA (translation) ought to reduce all of the downstream deleterious effects of the protein that lead to the manifestations of HD. These strategies aimed at reducing mHTT expression are considered among the most promising emerging therapeutics to slow or prevent HD [43, 44]. Three broad approaches are under investigation to reduce mHTT expression: RNA interference using short interfering RNA, translational repression using single-stranded DNA-based antisense oligonucleotides, and transcriptional repression using zinc finger proteins [45]. Modulation of mHTT phosphorylation, chaperone upregulation, and autophagy enhancement represent attempts to alter cellular homeostasis to favor removal of mHTT. The complex metabolic derangements in HD remain under study, but no clear therapeutic strategy has yet emerged. Many other therapeutic approaches for HD not properly genetic-based are underway. However, while there are many potential targets, few are well-validated and many single studies of purported success have yet to be replicated, including the failure in human patients of any agent that has been beneficial in an HD mouse model [45]. However, in the near future, multiple agents designed specifically to target the known pathobiology of HD will be introduced with a reasonable expectation of success.

The Cytochrome P450 System in Neurodegenerative Diseases

Currently, the concept that interindividual differences in genetic variations may be responsible for interindividual differences in drug response is widely accepted and has been validated in many research settings [46–50]. Polymorphisms in the cytochrome P450 (CYP) gene superfamily are the

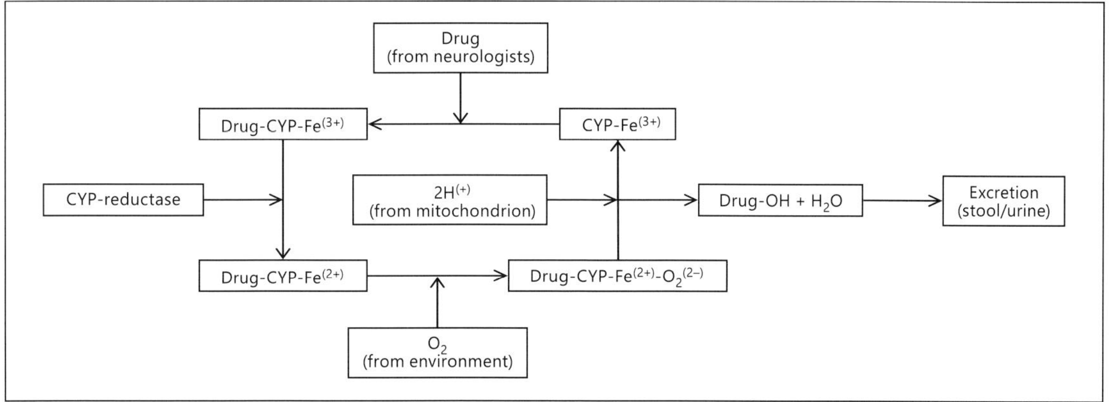

Fig. 1. Schematic representation of a CYP-mediated drug oxidation. The drug, a lipophilic compound, is converted into a more polar product readily excreted in stool and urine.

most important class of genetic factors influencing the response to treatment, and it is surprising that modern RCTs have not used this knowledge [51–53]. Currently, 18 CYP gene families and 44 CYP gene subfamilies have been described in humans, for a total of 9,000 CYP-named sequences [54–56], encoding enzymes with a catalytic activity potentially different from each other [57–59]. CYP enzymes are monooxygenases that catalyze an oxidative reaction, typically involving a substrate (the drug), a CYP reductase, and oxygen (fig. 1) [52, 53]. This rate of conversion is the key determinant of duration and intensity of drug efficacy. More than 90–95% of the CYP reactions with drugs are catalyzed only by 5 (CYP1A2, CYP2C9, CYP2C19, CYP2D6, and CYP3A4) of the 44 CYP subfamilies (11.36%), with the latter enzyme (CYP3A4) accounting for approximately 50% of the total CYP reactions [60].

Of closer relevance to neurodegenerative diseases is the use of tetrabenazine for the treatment of HD, whose dosing is based, only in part, on the CYP2D6 genotype [61] because the predictive value of this genotype is not high enough to accurately predict outcome by itself [62]. Also, the single nucleotide polymorphism rs1080985 in the CYP2D6 gene may influence the clinical efficacy of the AchEI donepezil in patients with mild-to-

moderate AD [63]. This finding has been replicated in an independent AD sample suggesting that this CYP2D6 variant might be useful as a predictor of poor response to short-term donepezil treatment [64]. The presence of gene variants conferring decreased or absent activity of the CYP2D6 enzyme was also significantly associated with a clinical response to donepezil treatment, suggesting that functional polymorphisms in the CYP2D6 gene can identify subgroups of patients with AD with different clinical responses to this drug [65]. Despite the need of a drug treatment for dementia with Lewy bodies and FTD spectrum, data regarding the use of AchEIs and other antidementia drugs in these neurodegenerative diseases are still valid. Thus, as well as for AD treatment, since rivastigmine and memantine are suicide substrates for diverse CYP (table 2), the concomitant use of drugs that are substrates for these CYP should be avoided.

Currently, the drugs with the strongest potential for pharmacogenetic recommendations in PD include benzatropine, L-DOPA, selegiline, ropinirole, cabergoline, rasagiline, bromocriptine, lisuride, and pergolide, and all are metabolized by CYP (table 3) with different action on the CYP enzyme activity. In particular, selegiline is a strong inhibitor of CYP2D6 and CYP2E1, and

Table 2. CYP-metabolized antidementia drugs

	CYP2A6	CYP2B6	CYP2C9	CYP2C19	CYP2D6	CYP3A4
Donepezil	–	–	S	–	S	S
Rivastigmine	–	–	–	–	Inh	Inh
Galantamine	–	–	–	–	S	S
Memantine	Inh	Inh	–	Inh	–	–

Inh = Inhibitor; S = substrate.

Table 3. CYP-metabolized drugs commonly used in the treatment of PD

	CYP1A2	CYP2A6	CYP2B6	CYP2C8	CYP2C9	CYP2C19	CYP2D6	CYP2E1	CYP3A4
Benzatropine	–	–	–	–	–	S	S	–	–
L-DOPA	–	–	–	–	–	–	S	–	–
Selegiline	S/Inh	S	S	S	S/Inh	S	Inh	Inh	S
Ropinirole	S/Inh	–	–	–	–	–	Inh		S
Cabergoline	–	–	–	–	–	–	–	–	S/Inh
Rasagiline	S	–	–	–	–	–	–	–	–
Bromocriptine	Inh	–	–	–	–	–	–	–	S/Inh
Lisuride	–	–	–	–	–	–	S	–	S
Pergolide	–	–	–	–	–	–	Inh	–	S/Inh

Inh = Inhibitor; S = substrate.

bromocriptine of CYP1A2, whereas ropinirole and pergolide are strong inhibitors of CYP2D6. Accordingly, the concomitant use of drugs that are substrates of these enzymes should be avoided. Evidence supporting the effect of substrates, inhibitors, or inducers of drug-specific metabolizing enzymes in anti-PD drug response also includes CYP1A2 in the response to ropinirole and rasagiline, and CYP3A4 in the response to bromocriptine, lisuride, pergolide, and cabergoline [66]. Notably, both entacapone and pramipexole are not CYP substrates. However, entacapone, a UDP-glucuronosyltransferase substrate, is a strong COMT (catechol O-methyltransferase) inhibitor [67]. Thus, the concomitant use of COMT drug substrates should be avoided. To sum up, there are no RCTs that take into account polymorphisms in drug metabolism enzymes in study design or analysis. In clinical practice, knowledge of variations in the activity of drug-metabolism enzymes and drug interactions could allow clinicians to choose the best therapeutic approach in terms of type of drug, drug association, and dosage.

Conclusions

Pharmacogenetics is founded on long-standing traditions in clinical practice, where therapies are selected based on history and physical findings in order to maximize benefit and minimize risks. Genetic tools allow increased sophistication in patient profiling and treatment optimization. Pharmaceutical companies are aware of the value of collecting genetic data during their RCTs.

Pharmacogenetic research is bidirectional with RCTs: efficacy data are correlated with genetic polymorphisms, which in turn define subjects for treatment stratification. The role of pharmacogenetics in RCTs for neurodegenerative diseases is still a young, unexplored, and promising field. A better understanding of the role of genetics in drug response to stratify patients in genetic homogeneous groups will have a great impact on RCT design, improving statistical power and allowing the identification of group-specific treatments. This will increase the success of phase III RCTs for therapeutic interventions in neurodegenerative diseases and will delineate the basis for future personalized medicine.

If it is true that RCTs must evaluate the efficacy of a given drug on a series of patients, it is also true that the role of genetics in influencing this response has been underestimated. It is clear that the great majority of neurodegenerative diseases are complex diseases in which genetic factors interact with nongenetic factors to produce clinical phenotypes. However, idiopathic PD, as well as AD, ALS, and other neurodegenerative diseases, have a strong genetic component [68] and RCTs ignore the role of genetics, which in turn leads to the failure of almost all RCTs in neurodegenerative diseases. Considering a clinical trial that is composed of a mixture of patients (as most are), some subjects may have a genotype that enables them to benefit from the drug, while others may have genotypes that make the drug ineffective or even harmful. By ignoring genetics, efficacy is measured on average, and the average may not be statistically significant, leading to the failure of the trial, with the result that a drug that might have helped a group of patients is abandoned. The FDA and the European Medicines Agency (EMA) have been promoting the application of pharmacogenetics in drug development for a decade, but in neurodegenerative diseases there still too few studies. In recent years, the complete characterization of the most important drug-metabolizing system has provided us with the knowledge to aim RCTs towards a second generation in which interindividual differences in drug metabolism do not bias the study, but instead become the basis to construct the trials, with the advantage of a cross-sectional role across diseases and drugs.

References

1 Panza F, Solfrizzi V, Imbimbo BP, Logroscino G: Amyloid-directed monoclonal antibodies for the treatment of Alzheimer's disease: the point of no return? Expert Opin Biol Ther 2014;14: 1465–1476.
2 Mahley RW, Weisgraber KH, Huang Y: Apolipoprotein E: structure determines function, from atherosclerosis to Alzheimer's disease to AIDS. J Lipid Res 2009;50(suppl):S183–S188.
3 Verghese PB, Castellano JM, Holtzman DM: Apolipoprotein E in Alzheimer's disease and other neurological disorders. Lancet Neurol 2011;10:241–252.
4 Rohrer JD, Guerreiro R, Vandrovcova J, et al: The heritability and genetics of frontotemporal lobar degeneration. Neurology 2009;73:1451–1456.
5 Rohrer JD, Warren JD: Phenotypic signatures of genetic frontotemporal dementia. Curr Opin Neurol 2011;24:542– 549.
6 Spatola M, Wider C: Genetics of Parkinson's disease: the yield. Parkinsonism Relat Disord 2014;20(suppl 1):S35–S38.
7 Morris JC, Aisen PS, Bateman RJ, et al: Developing an international network for Alzheimer research: the Dominantly Inherited Alzheimer Network. Clin Investig (Lond) 2012;2:975–984.
8 Panza F, Solfrizzi V, Imbimbo BP, Tortelli R, Santamato A, Logroscino G: Amyloid-based immunotherapy for Alzheimer's disease in the time of prevention trials: the way forward. Expert Rev Clin Immunol 2014;10:405– 419.
9 Lemere CA, Lopera F, Kosik KS, et al: The E280A presenilin 1 Alzheimer mutation produces increased Ab42 deposition and severe cerebellar pathology. Nat Med 1996;2:1146–1150.
10 Lopera F, Ardilla A, Martinez A, et al: Clinical features of early-onset Alzheimer disease in a large kindred with an E280A presenilin-1 mutation. JAMA 1997;277:793–799.
11 Reiman EM, Langbaum JB, Fleisher AS, et al: Alzheimer's Prevention Initiative: a plan to accelerate the evaluation of presymptomatic treatments. J Alzheimers Dis 2011;26(suppl 3):321–329.
12 Saunders AM, Strittmatter WJ, Schmechel D, et al: Association of apolipoprotein E allele epsilon 4 with late-onset familial and sporadic Alzheimer's disease. Neurology 1993;43:1467–1472.

13 Corder EH, Saunders AM, Strittmatter WJ, et al: Gene dose of apolipoprotein E type 4 allele and the risk of Alzheimer's disease in late onset families. Science 1993;261:921–923.

14 Farlow MR, Lahiri DK, Poirier J, Davignon J, Hui S: Apolipoprotein E genotype and gender influence response to tacrine therapy. NY Acad Sci 1996;802:101–110.

15 Farlow MR, Cyrus PA, Nadel A, Lahiri DK, Brashear A, Gulanski B: Metrifonate treatment of AD: influence of APOE genotype. Neurology 1999;53:2010–2016.

16 Farlow M, Lane R, Kudaravalli S, He Y: Differential qualitative responses to rivastigmine in APOE epsilon 4 carriers and noncarriers. Pharmacogenomics J 2004;4:332–335.

17 Suh GH, Jung HY, Lee CU, et al: Effect of the apolipoprotein E epsilon4 allele on the efficacy and tolerability of galantamine in the treatment of Alzheimer's disease. Dement Geriatr Cogn Disord 2006;21:33–39.

18 Risner ME, Saunders AM, Altman JF, et al; Rosiglitazone in Alzheimer's Disease Study Group: Efficacy of rosiglitazone in a genetically defined population with mild-to-moderate Alzheimer's disease. Pharmacogenomics J 2006;6:246–254.

19 Gold M, Alderton C, Zvartau-Hind M, et al: Rosiglitazone monotherapy in mild-to-moderate Alzheimer's disease: results from a randomized, double-blind, placebo-controlled phase III study. Dement Geriatr Cogn Disord 2010;30:131–146.

20 Salloway S, Sperling R, Gilman S, et al; Bapineuzumab 201 Clinical Trial Investigators: A phase 2 multiple ascending dose trial of bapineuzumab in mild to moderate Alzheimer disease. Neurology 2009;73:2061–2070.

21 Salloway S, Sperling R, Fox NC, et al: Two phase 3 trials of bapineuzumab in mild-to-moderate Alzheimer's disease. N Engl J Med 2014;370:322–333.

22 Reitz C, Mayeux R: Endophenotypes in normal brain morphology and Alzheimer's disease: a review. Neuroscience 2009;164:174–190.

23 Yu CE, Seltman H, Peskind ER, et al: Comprehensive analysis of APOE and selected proximate markers for late-onset Alzheimer's disease: patterns of linkage disequilibrium and disease/marker association. Genomics 2007;89:655–665.

24 Roses AD, Lutz MW, Amrine-Madsen H, et al: A TOMM40 variable-length polymorphism predicts the age of late-onset Alzheimer's disease. Pharmacogenomics J 2010;10:375–384.

25 Roses AD, Saunders AM, Lutz MW, et al: New applications of disease genetics and pharmacogenetics to drug development. Curr Opin Pharmacol 2014;14:81–89.

26 Crenshaw DG, Gottschalk WK, Lutz MW, et al: Using genetics to enable studies on the prevention of Alzheimer's disease. Clin Pharmacol Ther 2013;93:177–185.

27 Seelaar H, Rohrer JD, Pijnenburg YAL, Fox NC, van Swieten JC: Clinical, genetic and pathological heterogeneity of frontotemporal dementia: a review. J Neurol Neurosurg Psychiatry 2011;82:476–486.

28 Rohrer JD, Warren JD: Phenotypic signatures of genetic frontotemporal dementia. Curr Opin Neurol 2011;24:542–549.

29 Renton AE, Majounie E, Waite A, et al: A hexanucleotide repeat expansion in C9ORF72 is the cause of chromosome 9p21-linked ALS-FTD. Neuron 2011;72:257–268.

30 DeJesus-Hernandez M, Mackenzie IR, Boeve BF, et al: Rademakers R. Expanded GGGGCC hexanucleotide repeat in noncoding region of C9ORF72 causes chromosome 9p-linked FTD and ALS. Neuron 2011;72:245–256.

31 Borroni B, Alberici A, Cercignani M, et al: Granulin mutation drives brain damage and reorganization from preclinical to symptomatic FTLD. Neurobiol Aging 2012;33:2506–2520.

32 Ghidoni R, Stoppani E, Rossi G, et al: Optimal plasma progranulin cutoff value for predicting null progranulin mutations in neurodegenerative diseases: a multicenter Italian study. Neurodegener Dis 2012;9:121–127.

33 Capell A, Liebscher S, Fellerer K, et al: Rescue of progranulin deficiency associated with frontotemporal lobar degeneration by alkalizing reagents and inhibition of vacuolar ATPase. J Neurosci 2011;31:1885–1894.

34 Cenik B, Sephton CF, Dewey CM, et al: Suberoylanilide hydroxamic acid (Vorinostat) up-regulates progranulin transcription: rational therapeutic approach to frontotemporal dementia. J Biol Chem 2011;286:16101–16108.

35 Elamin M, Bede P, Byrne S, et al: Cognitive changes predict functional decline in ALS: a population-based longitudinal study. Neurology 2013;80:1590–1597.

36 Nicholson KA, Cudkowicz ME, Berry JD: Clinical trial designs in amyotrophic lateral sclerosis: does one design fit all? Neurotherapeutics 2015;12:376–383.

37 Miller TM, Pestronk A, DavidW, et al: An antisense oligonucleotide against SOD1 delivered intrathecally for patients with SOD1 familial amyotrophic lateral sclerosis: a phase 1, randomised, first-in-man study. Lancet Neurol 2013;12:435–442.

38 Perrin S: Preclinical research: make mouse studies work. Nature 2014;507:423–425.

39 Payami H, Factor SA: Promise of pharmacogenomics for drug discovery, treatment and prevention of Parkinson's disease. A perspective. Neurotherapeutics 2014;11:111–116.

40 Hamza TH, Chen H, Hill-Burns EM, et al: Genome-wide gene environment study identifies glutamate receptor gene GRIN2A as a Parkinson's disease modifier gene via interaction with coffee. PLoS Genet 2011;7:e1002237.

41 Hill-Burns EM, Singh N, Ganguly P, et al: A genetic basis for the variable effect of smoking/nicotine on Parkinson's disease. Pharmacogenomics J 2013;13:530–537.

42 Ross CA, Tabrizi SJ: Huntington's disease: from molecular pathogenesis to clinical treatment. Lancet Neurol 2011;10:83–98.

43 Magen I, Hornstein E: Oligonucleotide-based therapy for neurodegenerative diseases. Brain Res 2014;1584:116–128.

44 Garriga-Canut M, Agustín-Pavón C, Herrmann F, et al: Synthetic zinc finger repressors reduce mutant huntingtin expression in the brain of R6/2 mice. Proc Natl Acad Sci USA 2012;109:E3136–E3145.

45 Wild EJ, Tabrizi SJ: Targets for future clinical trials in Huntington's disease: what's in the pipeline? Mov Disord 2014;29:1434–1445.

46 Meyer UA: Pharmacogenetics and adverse drug reactions. Lancet 2000;356:1667–1671.

47 Pirmohamed M, Park BK: Genetic susceptibility to adverse drug reactions. Trends Pharmacol Sci 2001;22:298–305.

48 Güzey C, Spigset O: Genotyping as a tool to predict adverse drug reactions. Curr Top Med Chem 2004;4:1411–1421.

49 Wilke RA, Lin DW, Roden DM, et al: Identifying genetic risk factors for serious adverse drug reactions: current progress and challenges. Nat Rev Drug Discov 2007;6:904–916.

50 Ingelman-Sundberg M: Pharmacogenomic biomarkers for prediction of severe adverse drug reactions. N Engl J Med 2008;358:637–639.

51 Lynch T, Price A: The effect of cytochrome P450 metabolism on drug response, interactions, and adverse effects. Am Fam Physician 2007;76:391–396.

52 Seripa D, Pilotto A, Panza F, Matera MG, Pilotto A: Pharmacogenetics of cytochrome P450 (CYP) in the elderly. Ageing Res Rev 2010;9:457–474.

53 Johansson I, Ingelman-Sundberg M: Genetic polymorphism and toxicology – with emphasis on cytochrome p450. Toxicol Sci 2011;120:1–13.

54 Molecular basis of disease. Cytochrome P450s in humans. http://drnelson.uthsc.edu/P450.talks.html.

55 Sim SC, Ingelman-Sundberg M: The human cytochrome P450 Allele Nomenclature Committee web site: submission criteria, procedures, and objectives. Methods Mol Biol 2006;320:183–191.

56 The Human Cytochrome P450 (CYP) Allele Nomenclature Database. Allele nomenclature for Cytochrome P450 enzymes. http://www.cypalleles.ki.se/.

57 Ingelman-Sundberg M, Oscarson M, McLellan RA: Polymorphic human cytochrome P450 enzymes: an opportunity for individualized drug treatment. Trends Pharmacol Sci 1999;20:342–349.

58 Daly AK, Cholerton S, Gregory W, Idle JR: Metabolic polymorphisms. Pharmacol Ther 1993;57:129–160.

59 Evans WE, Relling MV: Pharmacogenomics: translating functional genomics into rational therapeutics. Science 1999;286:487–491.

60 Gardiner SJ, Begg EJ: Pharmacogenetics, drug-metabolizing enzymes, and clinical practice. Pharmacol Rev 2006;58:521–590.

61 Guay DR: Tetrabenazine, a monoamine-depleting drug used in the treatment of hyperkinetic movement disorders. Am J Geriatr Pharmacother 2010;8:331–373.

62 Mehanna R, Hunter C, Davidson A, Jimenez-Shahed J, Jankovic J: Analysis of CYP2D6 genotype and response to tetrabenazine. Mov Disord 2013;28:210–215.

63 Pilotto A, Franceschi M, D'Onofrio G, et al: Effect of a CYP2D6 polymorphism on the efficacy of donepezil in patients with Alzheimer disease. Neurology 2009;73:761–767.

64 Albani D, Martinelli Boneschi F, Biella G, et al: Replication study to confirm the role of CYP2D6 polymorphism rs1080985 on donepezil efficacy in Alzheimer's disease patients. J Alzheimers Dis 2012;30:745–749.

65 Seripa D, Bizzarro A, Pilotto A, et al: Role of cytochrome P4502D6 functional polymorphisms in the efficacy of donepezil in patients with Alzheimer's disease. Pharmacogenet Genomics 2011;21:225–230.

66 Agúndez JA, García-Martín E, Alonso-Navarro H, Jiménez-Jiménez FJ: Anti-Parkinson's disease drugs and pharmacogenetic considerations. Expert Opin Drug Metab Toxicol 2013;9:859–874.

67 Law V, Knox C, Djoumbou Y, et al: Drug Bank 4.0: shedding new light on drug metabolism. Nucleic Acids Res 2014;42:D1091–D1097.

68 Satake W, Nakabayashi Y, Mizuta I, et al: Genome-wide association study identifies common variants at four loci as genetic risk factors for Parkinson's disease. Nat Genet 2009;41:1303–1307.

Dr. Giancarlo Logroscino, MD, PhD
Unit of Neurodegenerative Diseases, Department of Clinical Research in Neurology
University of Bari 'Aldo Moro', 'Pia, Fondazione Cardinale G. Panico'
Via San Pio X n. 4
IT–73039 Tricase (Italy)
E-Mail giancarlo.logroscino@uniba.it

Beghi E, Logroscino G (eds): The Right Therapy for Neurological Disorders. From Randomized Trials to Clinical Practice.
Front Neurol Neurosci. Basel, Karger, 2016, vol 39, pp 136–146 (DOI: 10.1159/000445454)

Randomized Trials in Developing Countries: Different Priorities and Study Design?

Benoît Marin[a, b] · Gino Cédric Agbota[a, b] · Pierre-Marie Preux[a, b] · Farid Boumédiene[a, b]

[a]Inserm U1094, Tropical Neuroepidemiology, and [b]University of Limoges, UMR_S 1094, Tropical Neuroepidemiology, Institute of Neuroepidemiology and Tropical Neurology, CNRS FR 3503 GEIST, Limoges, France

Abstract

Background: Clinical trials are increasingly conducted in the field of neurology in developing countries. To our knowledge, no review has been performed to date about the temporal evolution, geographical distribution, pathological fields, and types of trials conducted. Besides, the validity of those clinical trials needs to be evaluated. ***Summary:*** Our main aim was to describe, using a systematic literature review, the clinical trials performed in the field of neurology in developing countries. The specific objectives were (1) to describe the pathologic fields, (2) to evaluate the methodology, and (3) to assess the validity of neurological clinical trials performed in developing countries. A systematic review of the literature was conducted accessing PubMed, Pascal, ScienceDirect, African Journal Online, and the Virtual Library of African Neurology. The 145 studies included allowed us to identify (1) an exponential evolution of the number of clinical trials, (2) the strong contributions from Asia, followed by Africa and Latin America, (3) a fairly good coverage of pathologic fields including noncommunicable diseases, (4) an increasing diversity of intervention type, (5) the lack of early-phase trials (phases I and IIa), and (5) the need of improvement for some critical methodological issues. ***Key Message:*** There is a need (1) to develop structures dedicated to the early investigation of interventions in humans, and (2) for sustaining the development of structures specialized in the methodology of clinical research and of dedicated courses for researchers in tropical areas about good practice in clinical trials. This would help in improving methodological quality, appropriateness of data management, and statistical analysis.

Clinical trials are experimental studies conducted with the participation of humans for the purpose of developing and improving the biological and medical knowledge on treatments or strategies. Clinical trials of drugs are performed to collect data on safety and tolerability, pharmacokinetics, pharmacodynamics, mechanisms of action, and efficacy of an experimental treatment.

The conduction of clinical trials is highly regulated. Since 1964, the World Medical Association has been gathering ethical principles within the Helsinki Declaration [1], which has been revised in subsequent years, especially in 2000. Likewise, based on this statement, guidelines of good practice in clinical trials (Good Clinical Practice) were developed in 1995 by the World Health Organization (WHO) [2] to ensure the rights, protection, well-being, and safety of participants in clinical trials.

Previously, clinical trials were conducted only in industrialized countries, mainly in Europe and the United States. They are now globalized and therefore done in developed countries as well as in developing countries.

While focusing on neurological diseases that can occur in tropical countries, it is possible to divide them into three main types. One type is neurological diseases seen in temperate regions and found in tropical areas: stroke, epilepsy, Alzheimer's disease, Parkinson's disease, bacterial meningitis, neurosyphilis, and multiple sclerosis. Another type is neurological diseases found predominantly or exclusively in tropical areas: cerebral malaria, tuberculosis meningitis, neurocysticercosis, and leprosy. Finally, the third type is tropical diseases with secondary damage to the nervous system: leptospirosis, schistosomiasis, trypanosomiasis, and trichinosis.

Tropical neurological disorders include some diseases that can be found everywhere, but for some of them the frequency is much higher in the tropics. For example, the overall prevalence of epilepsy given by African door-to door surveys is up to 13/1,000 compared to 5 per 1,000 in Western countries [3, 4].

Recent years have seen major advances in neurosciences and in particular tropical neurology for the treatment of certain conditions and for the identification of the relationships between infectious diseases and neurological disorders, such as the link between epilepsy and cerebral malaria [5–7]. Clinical trials are increasingly being conducted in the field of neurology in developing countries. This could be related to the reduction of cost of clinical trials in developing countries and the strong motivation of people who have access to free treatment. In addition, these people are often naive to any treatment, making them 'good subjects' for clinical research. However, it should be noted that the rather flexible regulation in developing countries may lead to clinical trials conducted with simplified procedures that are less stringent and secure [8, 9]. This raises the question of the validity of clinical trials in developing countries.

Our main aim was to describe, using a systematic literature review, the clinical trials that have been performed to date in the field of neurology in developing countries. The specific objectives were to describe the pathologic fields (1) to evaluate the methodology and then (2) to assess the validity of neurological clinical trials performed in developing countries.

Methods

Definitions

A *clinical trial* is an experiment (or intervention) conducted in humans in which participants are allocated to a health intervention in order to evaluate its efficacy or tolerability. Interventions include drugs, cells, and other biological products; surgical procedures; radiologic procedures; medical devices; behavioral treatments; adaptation to treatment protocols, and preventive care. This definition includes phase I–III trials.

To define *developing countries*, we used the classification from the World Bank based on gross national income per capita to identify 'developing countries' as those that are low-income and middle-income countries [10].

Search Strategy

The search was unlimited regarding the date of publication, but was restricted to articles in English. The following databases were searched through April 2014: PubMed (MEDLINE), Scopus, Pascal, ScienceDirect (Elsevier), African Journal Online, and the Virtual Library of African Neurology [Bibliothèque Virtuelle de Neurologie Africaine (BVNA)] which was created in 1982 and since then maintained by the Institute of Neuroepidemiology and Tropical Neurology of Limoges. It gathers articles published in African journals not indexed in popular databases (http://www.unilim.fr/ient/base-biblio-ient/). The keywords consisted of a

Table 1. Text words for the literature search

For clinical trials	'Clinical Trial, Phase I' [Publication Type] OR 'Clinical Trial, Phase II' [Publication Type] OR 'Clinical Trial, Phase III' [Publication Type] OR 'Pragmatic Clinical Trial' [Publication Type] OR 'Controlled Clinical Trial' [Publication Type] OR 'Randomized Controlled Trial' [Publication Type]
For neurology	'Neurology' [MeSH] OR 'Nervous system diseases' [MeSH]
For geographical areas	'Africa' [MeSH] OR 'Latin America' [MeSH] OR 'Central America' [MeSH] OR 'South America' [MeSH] OR 'Asia, Western' [MeSH] OR 'Asia, Southeastern' [MeSH] OR 'developing countries' [MeSH]

combination of medical subject headings (MeSH) and text words (table 1). All reports identified as relevant were imported into the bibliographic management tool Zotero and duplicates were deleted.

Inclusion Criteria
We included all original reports of clinical trials (phases I–III) focused on neurology (diseases of the central and peripheral nervous system) and conducted in a developing country. The following were excluded: (1) meta-analyses and literature reviews of epidemiological studies, (2) editorials and letters to the editor, (3) works in vitro and in vivo on animal or cell models, and (4) proceedings of conferences.

Study Selection
First, all titles were examined and some reports were excluded based on our selection criteria (stage 1). Second, abstracts were read (stage 2). These steps were performed by one author (G.C.A.) and validated by another (P.M.P.). Third, full texts of reports that complied with the inclusion criteria were examined (stage 3).

Data Extraction
One reviewer, who assessed their eligibility and extracted data, examined full copies of all selected reports. Data were recorded using an ad hoc form allowing collection of information about the study and elements to further ascertain the level of quality of the study included. The ICD-10 codes were used to classify the underlying disease [11]. Continent and subcontinent classification is based on those originated from the United Nations [12].

Ascertainment of Study Methodology
We used a grid for critical appraisal of the literature (table 2) based on that given by Salmi [13].

Results

Of 1,789 articles identified in the preliminary search, 302 were duplicates. After comprehensive screening (title, abstract), 1,274 references were excluded, leaving 213 relevant full texts. After examination of all full texts, 68 additional articles were excluded. Hence, 145 studies were included in the review. Figure 1 shows the flowchart of data selection for analysis.

Temporal Evolution and Geographical Distribution
Over a 40-year period, an exponential increase in the number of published studies was identified: 1% of studies (n = 1) were published between 1974 and 1984; 7% (n = 10) between 1984 and 1994; 28% (n = 40) between 1994 and 2004, and 64% (n = 94) between 2004 and 2014. These works originated from Asia (48.2%), Africa (35.9%), and Latin America (15.9%; fig. 2). 90% of studies from Asia were published before 2000 as compared to 73 and 74% from African and Latin American countries (p = 0.03). Africa was mostly represented by Western Africa (n = 24), Eastern Africa (n = 12), and Northern Africa (n = 4). Data from Asia

Disease: 10th ICM
Location: continent, country, region
Clear main objective: Y/N
Hypothesis stated: Y/N/NS
Sample size:
    Calculation of the sample size: Y/N/NS
    Appropriated sample size: Y/N/NS
Participants:
    Eligibility criteria given: Y/N/NS
    Patients able to receive both strategies: Y/N/NS/NA
    Appropriate duration of treatment and follow-up: Y/N/NS/NA
Interventions
    Precise definition: Y/N/NS
    Type of intervention: screening, prevention, diagnostic, therapeutic, rehabilitation, education
Main outcome accurate and reliable: Y/N/NS

Characteristics of the clinical trial
    Phase: I, II (a or b), III
    Design: parallel, cross-over, sequential, factorial
    Randomization: Y/N/NA
    Efficacy or noninferiority or equivalence
    Blinding: none, simple, double, triple
    Randomization performed by an independent unit: Y/N/NS
    Type of analysis: ITT/PP/NS
Ethical aspects
    Ethic committee approval: Y/N/NS
    Informed consent: Y/N/NS
Main results presented: Y/N
Discussion:
    Interpretation of the results: Y/N
    Overall proof: Y/N/NS
    Discussion about potential limitation: Y/N
Conclusion about validity of the study[1]: good[2], fair[3], acceptable[4], unacceptable[5]

Y = Yes; N = no; NA = not applicable; NS = not said; ITT = intent to treat; PP = per protocol; ICD = international classification of diseases. [1] Synthesis of the level of quality of the studies. [2] A study with at most 2 'no' or 'not said' answers for criteria that are not in italics as regards sample size, participants, study characteristics, discussion. [3] A study with 3–5 'no' or 'not said' answers for criteria that are not in italics as regards sample size, participants, study characteristics, discussion. [4] A study whose characteristics are not fully explained, i.e. at least 6 'no' or 'not said' answers for criteria that are not in italics as regards sample size, participants, study characteristics, discussion. [5] At least one 'no' answer for a criteria in italics.

originated from Central and Southern Asia (n = 43), Southeast Asia (n = 21), and East Asia (n = 6).

Pathological Fields

Most studies focused on infectious diseases (48%, n = 70), i.e. meningitis (n = 30), cerebral malaria (n = 18), poliomyelitis (n = 11), and neurocysticercosis (n = 7). Paroxysmal diseases were addressed in 25% of studies (n = 36). These included epilepsy (n = 12), stroke (n = 10), migraine (n = 8), convulsions (n = 4), and other (n = 2). Other diseases (27%, n = 39) were represented by neurodegenerative disorders (n = 5), neuromuscular disorders (n = 7), demyelinating disorders (n = 4), peripheral neuropathies (n = 7), cerebral palsy (n = 6), and other (n = 10).

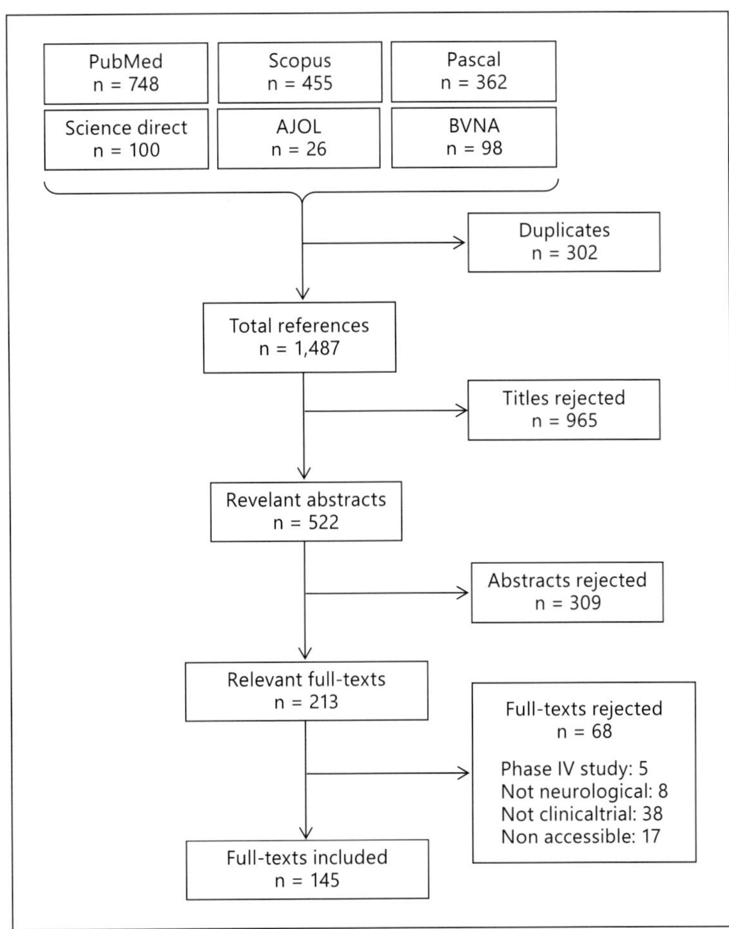

Fig. 1. Flowchart of eligibility criteria of the references. AJOL = African Journal Online.

In 67% of cases, studies from Africa focused on infectious diseases versus 41% from Asia and 27% from Latin America (p = 0.008). We identified a dramatic evolution over time of the distribution of pathological fields covered (i.e. before vs. after 2000; p = 0.02). While paroxysmal diseases represented respectively 22.2 and 25.4% in these periods, the proportion of the other diseases rose from 7.4 to 31.4% and the proportion of infectious diseases changed from 43.2 to 70.4%.

Methodological Characteristics

Phase III studies represented 84.1% (n = 122) versus 15.9% for phase II studies (n = 23). We did not identify any difference in the type of phase by continent (p = 0.15), but there was a difference with time, as 91.3% of phase II trials were published within the last 10 years versus 60.0% of phase III trials (p = 0.001).

These studies were focused on therapeutic (71.7%, n = 104), preventive (17.3%, n = 25), rehabilitative (10.3%, n = 15), and diagnostic interventions (0.7%, n = 1). Their distribution was not significantly different across continents (p = 0.56); however, we identified an evolution with time, as 93.3 and 80.0% of rehabilitative and preventive interventions, respectively, were published in the last 10 years as compared to 56.7% for therapeutic interventions (p = 0.02).

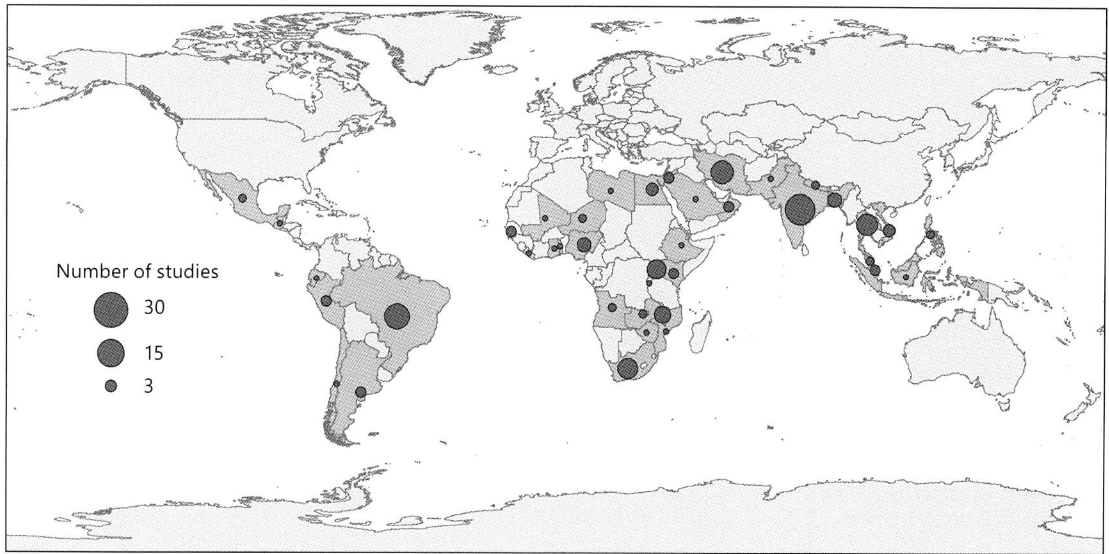

Fig. 2. Geographical distribution of neurological clinical trials performed in developing countries (n = 145).

Methodological Quality

The critical appraisal of the reports included in this review is presented in table 3. All articles clearly displayed the objectives, inclusion criteria, and definition of the condition and of the intervention. In all cases an accurate primary outcome was used. The research hypothesis was present in 85% of cases and a sample size calculation was available in 44.0% of studies. Randomization was clearly defined as performed by an independent center in only 11.0% of cases and analysis was clearly stated as done on an intent-to-treat basis in 31.0% of cases. Overall ethical aspects were satisfactory in 97.2% of studies, with ethical committee authorization and informed consent obtained from patients in 97.2%.

With time it was possible to observe significant improvement in the proportion of reports with sample size calculations (p = 0.03), respecting the ambivalence principle (p = 0.003), ethical committee authorizations (p = 0.02), informed consent (p = 0.02), and discussion of the limits of the study (p = 0.02). Based on these elements, 88% of studies were well conducted (33% good level,

48% fair level, 7% acceptable level) and 12% were of poor quality. Based on the evolution with time that was previously reported, an improvement of the quality was also identified with 25.6 versus 8.5% of inadequate quality before/after 2000 (p = 0.02). We did not identify differences in the quality of studies by continent.

Discussion

Geographical and Temporal Evolution

The results of this work show, over a 40-year period, an exponential increase in the number of published clinical trials that were performed on neurological disorders. The thematic fields that were addressed are quite large. Studies were mostly focused on the main infectious diseases occurring in tropical countries, such as meningitis, cerebral malaria, poliomyelitis, and neurocysticercosis. Nevertheless, there has been a progressive increase in the number of trials focused on paroxysmal disorders or other fields, for example neurodegenerative and neuromuscular

Table 3. Methodological characteristics of the included studies

Items	Overall	Before 2000	After 2000	p value
Presentation of objectives				
Yes	145 (100.0)	27 (18.6)	118 (81.4)	n.d.
No		0 (0.0)	0 (0.0)	
Presentation of hypothesis				
Yes	123 (84.8)	21 (77.8)	102 (86.4)	0.25
No	22 (15.2)	6 (22.2)	16 (13.6)	
Sample size calculation				
Yes	64 (44.1)	7 (25.9)	57 (48.3)	0.03
No	81 (55.9)	20 (74.1)	61 (51.7)	
Appropriate sample size				
Yes	97 (66.9)	17 (63.0)	80 (67.8)	0.84
No	13 (9.0)	3 (11.1)	10 (8.5)	
Unknown	35 (24.1)	7 (25.9)	28 (23.7)	
Presentation of eligibility criteria				
Yes	145 (100.0)	27 (100.0)	118 (100.0)	n.d.
No	0 (0.0)	0 (0.0)	0 (0.0)	
Patients able to receive both strategies				
Yes	116 (80.0)	13 (48.1)	103 (87.3)	0.003
No	1 (0.7)	0 (0.0)	1 (0.8)	
Unknown	28 (19.3)	14 (51.8)	14 (11.8)	
Appropriate length of follow-up				
Yes	139 (95.8)	26 (96.3)	113 (95.8)	1
No	1 (0.7)	0 (0.0)	1 (0.1)	
Unknown	5 (3.4)	1 (3.7)	4 (3.4)	
Definition of type of intervention				
Yes	145 (100.0)	27 (100.0)	118 (100.0)	n.d.
No		0 (0.0)	0 (0.0)	
Type of intervention				
Therapeutic	104 (71.7)	23 (85.2)	81 (68.6)	0.17
Preventive	25 (17.2)	4 (14.8)	21 (17.8)	
Rehabilitative	15 (6.9)	0 (0)	15 (12.7)	
Diagnostic	1 (0.7)	0 (0)	1 (0.9)	
Phase				
II	23 (15.9)	2 (7.4)	21 (17.8)	0.25
III	122 (84.1)	25 (92.6)	97 (82.2)	
Design				
Parallel	141 (97.2)	27 (100.0)	114 (96.6)	1
Cross-over	2 (1.4)	0 (0.0)	2 (0.0)	
Factorial	2 (1.4)	0 (0.0)	2 (0.0)	
Randomization				
Yes	142 (97.9)	27 (100.00)	115 (97.4)	1
No	3 (2.1)	0 (0)	3 (2.6)	
Perspective				
Efficacy	134 (92.4)	25 (92.6)	109 (92.4)	1
Noninferiority	11 (7.6)	2 (7.4)	9 (7.6)	
Blinding				
No	73 (50)	17 (63.0)	56 (47.4)	0.51
Simple	16 (11)	1 (3.7)	15 (12.7)	
Double	52 (36)	9 (33.3)	43 (36.4)	
Triple	1 (0.7)	0 (0.0)	1 (100)	
Not applicable	3 (2.5)	0 (0.0)	3 (100)	

Items	Overall	Before 2000	After 2000	p value
Randomization by an independent center				
Yes	16 (11.0)	1 (3.7)	15 (12.7)	0.37
No	121 (83.4)	26 (96.3)	95 (80.5)	
Unknown	5 (3.4)	0 (0.0)	5 (4.2)	
Not applicable	3 (2.1)	0 (0.0)	3 (2.5)	
Analysis				
Intent-to-treat	45 (31.0)	4 (14.8)	41 (34.7)	0.10[1]
Per protocol	3 (2.1)	0 (0.0)	3 (2.5)	
Unknown	97 (67.0)	23 (85.1)	74 (62.7)	
Appropriate, accurate and reliable main outcome				
Yes	145 (100.0)	27 (100.0)	118 (100.0)	n.d.
No	0 (0.0)	0 (0.0)	0 (0.0)	
Ethical committee				
Yes	141 (97.2)	24 (88.9)	117 (99.2)	0.02
Unknown	4 (2.8)	3 (11.1)	1 (0.8)	
Obtention of an informed consent				
Yes	141 (97.2)	24 (88.9)	117 (99.1)	0.02
No	4 (2.7)	3 (11.1)	1 (0.9)	
Presentation of main results				
Yes	145 (100)	27 (100.0)	118 (100.0)	n.d.
No	0 (0.0)	0 (0.0)	0 (0.0)	
Interpretation of results				
Yes	145 (100.0)	27 (100.0)	118 (100.0)	n.d.
No	0 (0.0)	0 (0.0)	0 (0.0)	
Overall evidence				
Yes	117 (80.7)	22 (81.5)	95 (80.5)	0.91
No	28 (19.3)	5 (18.5)	23 (19.5)	
Discussion of limits				
Yes	43 (29.6)	3 (11.1)	40 (33.9)	0.02
No	102 (70.3)	24 (88.9)	78 (66.1)	
Conclusion				
Good	48 (33.1)	5 (18.5)	43 (36.4)	0.05
Fair	70 (48.2)	13 (48.2)	57 (50.0)	
Acceptable	10 (6.9)	2 (7.5)	8 (7.0)	
Inadequate	17 (11.7)	7 (2.6)	10 (8.8)	

Values are given as n (%). p value for comparison between before/after 2000, χ^2 or Fisher's exact test. n.d. = Not done. [1] In phase III only.

disorders. At the same time, the types of intervention have evolved with the recent development of studies focused on prevention and rehabilitation.

This review also documents the recent impulse of the Indian continent in the field of research, with 63 works published in the last 20 years (i.e. 41% of all studies included in our review). This is probably related to population growth, industrialization, and increase of the skills in research in this continent.

A Growing Number of Trials
The first observation of this work is the growing number of studies conducted in developing countries. This might be explained by socioeconomic

development in recent years, which has helped to generate more funding for research in general and for clinical research in particular. Economic improvement may also lead to an increase in the number of qualified human resources and of technical resources (clinical research centers, specialized laboratories, medical equipment), and then to the implementation of more specialized and more advanced studies in the medical field. The pharmaceutical industry could have also contributed to this growth in new target territories. Three points might also explain the attractiveness of developing countries for clinical research:

(1) Reduction of costs: compared to developed countries, the salary of the staff involved in a clinical study (doctor, nurse, and coordinator of the study) is lower. For example, the cost of a site investigator in India is 40–50% lower than in the United States [14].

(2) Easier recruitment of patients: it has been shown that the average number of patients per site in developing countries is up to 10 times higher than that of Western Europe [15]. This fact can be explained by a closer doctor/patient relationship, which results in less hesitation of the patients to follow the suggestions made by their doctors. This can also be explained by the existence of a large population of patients meeting the inclusion criteria for clinical trials (e.g. population naive of any treatment). Finally, for some populations, in the absence of public insurance systems and high health costs, the frame of a clinical trial might be the only possibility to receive a treatment. This latter point raises ethical concerns.

(3) A weaker regulatory environment: the regulatory environment in developing countries may be less strict than in developed countries. This flexibility might favor easier and faster implementation of clinical trials.

Pathological Fields

Clinical trials in developing countries have predominantly focused on therapeutic interventions and have been mainly targeted on infectious diseases. This result was expected, as the prevailing conditions in the tropics are infectious diseases.

In recent years, however, noncommunicable diseases (NCDs) have become the leading cause of morbidity and mortality in the world, including developing countries. According to the WHO, nearly 80% of deaths are due to NCDs worldwide. This works out to approximately 36 million deaths, of which 29 million occur in low- and middle-income countries. Also, 90% of 'premature' deaths due to NCDs are registered in low- and middle-income countries. According to the WHO, in the past decade and among NCDs, stroke was the second leading cause of death [16].

In this regard, one may wonder why NCDs are not the subject of more studies in developing countries. One might assume that the lack of technical resources (advanced laboratories, new analytical imaging methods, etc.) has an impact on the feasibility in the conduct of clinical trials in the field of NCDs [16, 17].

Phases of Clinical Trials and Needs

Clinical trials have been phases IIb and III. It seems that no phase I or IIa has been published in the field of neurology from developing countries. This finding may be explained by the lack of technical resources such as specialized laboratories and well-equipped resuscitation units, which are mandatory for the implementation of such clinical trials. Therapeutic phase I trials aim to assess tolerability versus dose and to make a pharmacokinetic profile and preliminary pharmacodynamics of the drug in humans. Phase IIa trials are designed to improve knowledge of the pharmacokinetics and pharmacodynamics in humans. These two early phases are essential to determine the safety and dosage of drugs. They are mainly conducted in the United States and Europe. Knowing that the tolerability of a drug may vary depending on population genetics, the assessment of safety and pharmacokinetic and pharmacodynamic properties of a drug only in one population may have relevant ethical implications. For example, carbamazepine, a drug with antiseizure properties for which phase I and II trials were performed in the United States and Europe, was subsequently assessed with phase III trials in Asia. While this molecule was well tolerated in Europe, it caused serious adverse reactions in Asia (Stevens-Johnson syndrome, necrotizing toxiderma) due to the genetic background of Asian subjects (HLA-B*1,502, HLA-B*1,518), resulting in altered metabolism of this molecule [18–20]. Hence, there is a need to develop structures dedicated to the early investigation of these aspects in humans in resource-poor countries.

Quality of Clinical Trials in Neurology and Needs
Overall, clinical trials in developing countries were conducted with a fairly appropriate methodology (88.0%), although only 33.1% of the studies reached the highest level of quality. Some elements need urgent improvements. It is indeed striking to identify such a low percentage of studies with appropriate sample size (66.9%), sample size calculation (44.0%), blinding (50.0), intent-to-treat analysis (31.0%), evaluation of the limits of the study (29.7%), and randomization by an independent center (11.0%). This reinforces the need for sustaining the development of dedicated courses for students and researchers in tropical areas about good practice in clinical trials. Furthermore, these elements plead for continuing the development of structures specialized in the methodology of clinical research in tropical

zones. This would help in increasing the level of methodological quality, appropriateness of data management, and statistical analysis.

Conclusion

The 145 studies included in this review allowed us to identify (1) an exponential increase in the number of clinical trials within the 40-year period investigated, (2) the strong contribution Asia (48.2% of studies), followed by Africa (35.9%) and Latin America (15.9), (3) a fairly good coverage of pathologic fields including infectious diseases as well as NCDs, (4) an increasing diversity of intervention types (preventive and rehabilitation studies), especially in the 10 last years, (5) the lack of early-phase trials (none in phase I or IIa), and (5) an overall appropriate methodology of the studies but the need for improvements of some critical methodological issues (process of randomization, sample size determination, blinding, intent-to-treat analysis).

These results highlight the need to develop highly equipped structures in tropical countries dedicated to the early investigation of interventions in humans in order to solve the lack of phase I or IIa studies. More globally, an effort should be made to organize and fund structures specialized in the methodology of clinical research in tropical areas. Local leaders need to face this priority. This would sustain the improvement of the methodological quality of all studies (at the same time helping local researchers in their careers) and reinforce the empowerment of tropical areas for the conduction of clinical trials.

References

1 Word Medical Association: Declaration of Helsinki – Ethical Principles for Medical Research Involving Human Subjects. http://www.wma.net/en/30publications/10policies/b3/index.html (accessed July 14, 2014).

2 European Medicines Agency: Note for guidance on good clinical practice (CPMP/ICH/135/95). http://ethikkommission.meduniwien.ac.at/fileadmin/ethik/media/dokumente/rechtsgrundlagen/GCP.pdf (accessed July 14, 2014).

3 Genton P, Remy C: L'épilepsie. Tours, Ellipse, 1996.

4   Ba-Diop A, Marin B, Druet-Cabanac M, Ngoungou EB, Newton CR, Preux PM: Epidemiology, causes, and treatment of epilepsy in sub-Saharan Africa. Lancet Neurol 2014;13:1029–1044.

5   Ngoungou EB, Preux PM: Cerebral malaria and epilepsy. Epilepsia 2008;49:19–24.

6   Ngoungou EB, Koko J, Druet-Cabanac M, et al: Cerebral malaria and sequelar epilepsy: first matched case-control study in Gabon. Epilepsia 2006;47:2147–2153.

7   Ngoungou EB, Dulac O, Poudiougou B, et al: Epilepsy as a consequence of cerebral malaria in area in which malaria is endemic in Mali, West Africa. Epilepsia 2006;47:873–879.

8   Chippaux JP: Pratique des essais cliniques en Afrique. Paris, IRD Editions, 2004.

9   Cot M: Should clinical research in developing countries be supported (in French)? Rev Epidemiol Sante Publique 2003;51:297–300.

10   World Bank: New country classification. http://data.worldbank.org/news/new-country-classifications (accessed July 14, 2014).

11   World Health Organization: International Statistical Classification of Diseases and Related Health Problems 10th Revision. http://apps.who.int/classifications/icd10/browse/2010/en (accessed July 14, 2014).

12   United Nations: Composition of macro geographical (continental) regions, geographical sub-regions, and selected economic and other groupings. http://unstats.un.org/unsd/methods/m49/m49regin.htm (accessed July 14, 2014).

13   Salmi LR: Lecture critique et rédaction médicale scientifique. Comment lire, rédiger et publier une étude clinique ou épidémiologique? Paris, Elsevier, 1998.

14   Garnier JP: Rebuilding the R&D engine in big pharma. Harv Bus Rev 2008;86:68–70, 72–76, 128.

15   Mathis G: Clinical trials in rapidly developing economies – what to look for, what to prepare for. J Clin Stud 2009, pp 44–45. https://mediciglobal.com/assets/docs/Survival_of_the_Fittest_Article_in_JCS_Jan_2009_pdf.pdf (accessed December 21, 2015).

16   World Health Organization: The top 10 causes of death. http://www.who.int/mediacentre/factsheets/fs310/en/ (accessed July 14, 2014).

17   World Health Organization: Noncommunicable diseases. http://www.who.int/mediacentre/factsheets/fs355/en/ (accessed July 14, 2014).

18   Hung SI, Chung WH, Jee SH, et al: Genetic susceptibility to carbamazepine-induced cutaneous adverse drug reactions. Pharmacogenet Genomics 2006;16:297–306.

19   Ikeda H, Takahashi Y, Yamazaki E, et al: HLA class I markers in Japanese patients with carbamazepine-induced cutaneous adverse reactions. Epilepsia 2010;51:297–300.

20   Yang CW, Hung SI, Juo CG, et al: HLA-B*1502-bound peptides: implications for the pathogenesis of carbamazepine-induced Stevens-Johnson syndrome. J Allergy Clin Immunol 2007;120:870–877.

Prof. Pierre Marie Preux
INSERM UMR1094, Tropical Neuroepidemiology, Institute of Neuroepidemiology and Tropical Neurology
School of Medicine, University of Limoges
2 rue du Dr Marcland
FR–87025 Limoges (France)
E-Mail preux@unilim.fr

Beghi E, Logroscino G (eds): The Right Therapy for Neurological Disorders. From Randomized Trials to Clinical Practice.
Front Neurol Neurosci. Basel, Karger, 2016, vol 39, pp 147–153 (DOI: 10.1159/000445455)

The Right Therapy for Neurological Disorders: From Randomized Trials to Clinical Practice – Patients versus Investigator Expectations and Needs

Lucie I. Bruijn[a] · Steve Kolb[b]

[a] ALS Association, Washington, D.C., and [b] Patient Advocat, Norfolk, Va., USA

Abstract

Background: People living with amyotrophic lateral sclerosis (ALS) are now more proactive in making decisions about their treatment options, in particular with increased awareness through social media and the Internet. Together with increased awareness about the disease comes increased frustration that there is still only one Food and Drug Administration (FDA)-approved drug that modestly improves survival. **Summary:** While efforts are underway to improve clinical trial design, patient involvement in trial design, clinical outcomes, and risk/benefit evaluations have become more recognized and will play a major role in the future success of clinical trials. This chapter addresses the perspective of people living with ALS and their perceptions of clinical trials. We describe various organizations and programs available that provide increased education and patient involvement. **Key Message:** Stronger partnerships between those living with ALS, clinicians, government, nonprofit organizations, and regulatory agencies will significantly impact treatment development. © 2016 S. Karger AG, Basel

In July and August 2014 we witnessed an unprecedented social media phenomenon which changed the amyotrophic lateral sclerosis (ALS)/motor neuron disease (MND) landscape in multiple ways. This transformation was led by Pat Quinn, Pete Frates (individuals living with ALS), and their families who are credited with taking the campaign viral in Massachusetts (USA) in mid-July 2014. People globally, many without any connection to the disease, participated in The ALS Ice Bucket Challenge. This brought exceptional awareness and increased revenue to ALS research and patient care, through contributions to numerous advocacy and research organizations. Paralleling this excitement was heightened frustration in the ALS community due to lack of treatments significantly altering the course of the disease. Despite advances in ALS research and dramatic improvements in clinical management, there is still only one drug, Rilutek, which modestly improves survival.

Patient frustration was illustrated most recently with the drug, GM604, also known as GM6, a compound that has received fast track and orphan drug designation from the US Food and Drug Administration (FDA) for the treatment of ALS. GM6 was tested in 12 people living with ALS (8 drug, 4 placebo) for 2 weeks and followed for an additional 10 weeks. The study was designed to test safety and tolerability in people with ALS and was reported by the company Genervon to show promise. In the absence of other new compounds showing benefit for ALS, the patient community, with the company's encouragement, has lobbied for accelerated approval of the compound. This coincides with many US states developing 'right to try' legislation which would make experimental drugs under review for approval at the FDA and that have passed initial toxicity and dosage testing (phase I) available to terminally ill patients, with the permission of their physician and the drug manufacturer. This reflects a lessening of concern among many ALS patients about potential risks posed by novel therapies and more determination to have immediate access to any treatment with perceived promise.

These recent events illustrate a changing perspective and role for those living with ALS in the clinical trials arena and should be considered as we move forward in developing future clinical trials. Significant efforts are underway to better inform the ALS community about the need for rigorous clinical trials; however, clinicians must increase patient engagement in research and clinical trials. This will have a significant impact on improving clinical trial design and trial enrolment. These efforts should be made in conjunction with close cooperation with the FDA and the European Medicines Agency (EMA).

Limitations of Clinical Trials from the Patient Perspective

For many living with the disease, enrolment in clinical trials provides a sense of hope. Of course, everyone hopes that the treatment under trial will benefit them, but many also derive satisfaction from the knowledge that, even if the treatment is not effective, the information gained will help others facing this terrible disease. Patients and their families are often frustrated if they are unable to participate in a trial due to its inclusion/exclusion criteria. This is particularly true for those who have a more slowly progressing form of the disease. The explanation that inclusion of these patients in the trial may lead to false-positive results is reasonable from a scientific standpoint, but difficult for patients and families to accept. An additional challenge is the need for control groups (who receive placebos) in clinical trials. Adaptive clinical trial designs are attempting to address this issue, including increased discussions about the use of historical controls. This topic remains controversial especially as studies have shown that improved care and clinical management over the past years have been shown to increase the survival of patients and could affect the trial results if not carefully controlled for in multicenter studies. These issues are particularly a concern in stem cell trials where invasive 'sham surgeries' are required to establish a control group, and this may be seen as unethical. Enrolment in ALS clinical trials featuring drugs already available for treatment of other diseases is also challenging because patients may choose to acquire the drug outside of the trial context, thus making the trial more difficult to populate.

There is a perception among many patients and families that the FDA significantly delays progress in clinical trials and access to treatment. While there are efforts underway to address areas which can benefit from improved interaction with the FDA, many programs already exist to incentivize companies to expedite treatment development for rare disease such as ALS. The technical challenges for bringing a new therapy to people with ALS are formidable. As a result, every effort needs to be made to improve and accelerate the drug development process. Regulatory requirements are a significant dimension of this effort and an area where the patient and caregiver perspective is increasingly important.

The Orphan Disease Act, passed in 1983, created financial incentives, including grants, to support the development of new drugs for people with rare diseases. Under this system, developers of promising drugs, including biologics, can apply to receive 'orphan designation'. Orphan designation provides financial incentives for the development of products for qualifying rare diseases.

Fast track designation is intended to facilitate the development and expedite the review of drugs to treat serious conditions and fill an unmet medical need. Designation may be granted on the basis of preclinical or clinical data. Fast track designation typically supports both early and more frequent interactions with the FDA during drug development. In addition, sponsors can submit portions of a fast track marketing application as they are ready and before submitting the complete application, using a practice that is known as 'rolling review'.

The accelerated approval pathway can be used to expedite the development and approval of promising therapies that treat a serious or life-threatening condition and provide meaningful therapeutic benefit over available therapies. Accelerated approval allows approval of a drug that demonstrates an effect on a 'surrogate end point' that is reasonably likely to predict clinical benefit, or on the basis of an effect on a clinical end point that can be measured earlier than the effect on survival or irreversible morbidity, which is reasonably likely to predict an effect on irreversible morbidity or mortality or other clinical benefit.

The FDA has long had in place a review system to ensure that the most critical medical products are reviewed on a priority basis. The goal for priority review applications for products that offer major advances in treatment, or provide a treatment when no adequate therapy exists, is to complete them within a 6-month period, compared to the 10-month goal for standard review of other products.

The FDA Safety and Innovation Act (FDA-SIA) also established another program that is intended to expedite the development and review of drugs for serious or life-threatening conditions, known as 'breakthrough therapy designation'. To obtain a breakthrough therapy designation, a drug must be intended to treat a serious or life-threatening condition, and preliminary clinical evidence must demonstrate that the drug may provide substantial improvement on at least one clinically significant end point over available therapy. A breakthrough therapy designation conveys all of the fast track program features, as well as more intensive FDA guidance for an efficient drug development program, including an organizational commitment to involve senior managers and experienced review staff.

In many rare diseases, ALS included, certain factors can be critical in the regulatory review process for candidate therapies such as a smaller number of patients for clinical trials, various disease mechanisms, patient-reported outcomes, and the benefit-risk profile of individuals with ALS. This can be facilitated by FDA guidance documents. These are official documents that explain the agency's interpretation of, or policy on, a regulatory issue. The FDA prepares guidances primarily for industry, but also for other stakeholders and its own staff, and uses them to address such matters as the design, manufacturing, and testing of regulated products; scientific issues; content and evaluation of applications for product approvals, and inspection and enforcement policies (http://www.fda.gov/downloads/AboutFDA/Transparency/Transparency Initiative/UCM285124.pdf).

Currently, there is no FDA Guidance specific to ALS product development that would address these issues for sponsors or other interested stakeholders. Such a document could significantly facilitate and speed ALS therapy development, as well as enhance the consistency and quality of the application review process, while also encouraging more industry partners to enter the field. A draft guidance document has been developed by the EMA as a guidance for the evaluation of drugs for the treatment of ALS. The guideline focuses on treatment aimed to modify disease progression (http://www.ema.europa.eu/docs/en_GB/document_library/Scientific_guideline/2013/07/WC500147005.pdf).

Recently, under a patient-focused drug development thrust, the FDA has been working to more deeply engage patients and stakeholders in the regulatory arena. A ground-breaking effort over the last year between the agency and the Duchenne muscular dystrophy community has demonstrated the opportunity for a patient advocacy organization to drive a collaborative improvement effort for a drug development guidance. This process will enable the FDA to approach the disease and candidate therapies with better understanding of the related issues and to expedite a specific guidance. Limited agency resources also mean that many potential guidance topics would not be addressed without this community leadership. A similar effort to draft a guidance document is currently being undertaken by the ALS community and working groups for biomarkers, clinical trial design, benefit/risk, clinical outcomes, public policy, and ALS and frontotemporal dementia. Once the externally prepared draft guidance material is submitted to the FDA, the agency will then move through its internal evaluation, draft development, public comment, and guidance finalization steps, which may incorporate all or some of the draft materials submitted by the ALS community.

Approaches to Improved Understanding of the Value of Clinical Trials and the Impact of Patient Engagement

Many ALS organizations, including The ALS Association, Muscular Dystrophy Association, and the Motor Neurone Disease Association

UK work closely with the clinical community to encourage enrolment into clinical trials, educate about the importance of clinical trials, and help the ALS community understand the challenges of 'overinterpreting' the efficacy of small trials.

The need to guide those with ALS/MND to reliable sources of web-based information was highlighted by Chen and Turner [1] in 2011, who note that access to the Internet can lead to misleading results, which can cause considerable problems for people affected by ALS/MND, particularly their children. As variable search terms can be used, with differing and unfiltered results, this can lead to false hope or inaccurate information, particularly if a child (or other family member) is trying to identify symptoms, treatments, and hoped for cures for a parent diagnosed with ALS.

The Internet is an incredible source of information (Landro [2] wrote an interesting article in the *Wall Street Journal* highlighting the 'clout' of online patient fora). Misinterpretation, however, of information gained through the Internet can easily lead to a breakdown in confidence between patient and clinician when possible 'cures' or 'treatments' are dismissed by the clinician.

PatientsLikeMe®

PatientsLikeMe® (www.patientslikeme.com) is a patient network aiming to improve lives and provide a real-time research platform for patient engagement. Through the network, patients connect with others who have the same disease or condition and track and share their own experiences. In the process, they generate data about the real-world nature of disease that help researchers, pharmaceutical companies, regulators, providers, and nonprofit organizations develop more effective products, services, and care. PatientsLikeMe has 325,000 members and partners with the pharmaceutical industry and academic institutions. Wicks et al. [3] argue the multiple benefits experienced by patients using sites such as PatientsLikeMe (which include peer to peer support through the online community) result in better management of symptom side effects. Additionally, the concentration of people internationally using the site has supported clinical research, such as that conducted by Chen and Turner [1], 2010, through an online survey of people with ALS/MND.

ALS Untangled

In the absence of traditional medicines to alter the trajectory of the disease, many ALS patients have turned to alternative and off-label options. These options are discussed widely among patients through social media.

ALS Untangled (http://www.alsuntangled. com/) brings a scientific review process to these nontraditional treatments. Treatments are selected based on patient input via Twitter, and reviewed according to various criteria, including the rationale behind the perceived mechanism, preclinical data (if any), and safety. Treatments are examined in order, based on the number of requests received for that particular option to be reviewed.

While the primary purpose of ALS Untangled is to discern possible treatment options, there may be an equally important gain for the community: patient empowerment. In a disease where so few options are available, patients often express a willingness to 'try anything that might work'. ALS Untangled gives them information to help guide their choices, sometimes born of frustration, and avoid options that may be detrimental to their health, or wasteful of financial resources.

Reviews include various nutritional supplements, 'natural' remedies (bee venom, coconut oil), and treatment protocols.

Clinical Research Learning Institute

The Clinical Research Learning Institute (CRLI) is a program of the Northeast ALS Consortium (NEALS) and funded by the ALS Association that is 'committed to educating patient-caregiver pairs on clinical research and therapy development in order to improve their ability to advocate locally and nationally for clinical research' [4]. These 2-day programs include in-depth training in current ALS treatment development, and exposure to the clinical trial process, including how to evaluate published trial results.

The Patient-Centered Outcomes Research Institute

Patients with ALS are the principal stakeholders with an interest in the development of biomarkers that are likely to aid therapeutic development. The Patient-Centered Outcomes Research Institute (PCORI) is a nonprofit, nongovernmental organization located in Washington, DC. Congress authorized the establishment of PCORI in the Patient Protection and Affordable Care Act of 2010, with the goal of supporting patient-centered research and infrastructure. Funding for Patient Powered Research Networks (PPRN) is one of the mechanisms PCORI uses to further the goal of patient-centered research.

Centre for the Advancement of Sustainable Medical Innovation

The Centre for the Advancement of Sustainable Medical Innovation (CASMI; http://casmi.org. uk/) is a partnership between Oxford University and UCL, created to develop new models for medical innovation. The center aims to address the issues that have led to current failures in the translation of basic bioscience into affordable and widely adopted new treatments. The center combines academically rigorous research with high-impact policy work. It brings together multiple disciplines and stakeholders to tackle major issues such as value, regulation, adherence, and the translation of advanced therapies. CASMI advises governments and other bodies on the relevant public policy and regulatory issues to stimulate and develop the life sciences sectors, and positions the patient perspective at the center of all their work.

How Can the ALS Trial Community Better Serve Patients?

At the same time as the trials community increases the rigor with which it approaches trial design, it should be careful not to lose focus on patient needs and experiences within the trial process. There are several potential areas for improvement. A significant opportunity lies in the development and expansion of telemedicine to clinical trials. Currently, patients wishing to participate in a trial usually must return to the clinical center for monitoring, entailing costs and inconvenience in the best of cases. In-home telemedicine visits, with caregivers trained to assist in administering the standard clinical measures used in trials, such as the ALS Functional Rating Scale (ALSFRS) and perhaps ventilatory function, are possible and may be practical for many trials, and would likely lower the barrier to enrolment, especially for patients who live far from their treatment center. This may be especially beneficial for nonintervention trials (i.e. those not testing a putative therapy), in which there is no potential for therapeutic improvement. Also, patients can and should be asked more often about which outcome measures would be most relevant to them; these are often quality-of-life end points, and incorporating them may increase patients' sense that the trial is focused on their needs, and may reveal treatment benefits that clinicians have previously overlooked.

Current regulations in all countries emphasize the paramount importance of establishing that humans will not be exposed to unreasonable risk before a new treatment can be tested in a clinical trial. While recognizing that importance, those affected by ALS often become frustrated with the pace of regulatory approval for new trials, making the argument that their disease is a more certain danger than a putative treatment is likely to be. There is no simple answer to balancing safety risks with the urgency of finding new therapies, but a recognition that patients may be willing to accept a higher level of risk may help clinical researchers and regulatory authorities as they examine risk/benefit calculations for new agents. At the same time, patients are often dismayed by the requirement for a placebo arm in drug trials, as it lowers the odds of receiving a potentially helpful new treatment.

One option proposed for reducing the size of the placebo arm in the earliest phases of development is to supplement it with data from historic controls. However, as discussed earlier, because of the evolving standard of care in ALS, data from older studies are unlikely to offer a valid comparison group for current trials. An alternative is to use a 2:1 ratio of active treatment to placebo. It is important to note that therapy development in general is accelerated by conducting well-designed studies, which include the use of appropriate controls. As was seen in the minocycline trial, some active treatments may be harmful, and patients in the placebo arm have a better outcome [5].

Whatever the specific trial design, clinicians have the obligation to take time to discuss with patients and families the reasons behind the structure of trials, including placebo arms, blinding, the primacy of safety, etc. Understanding the complexity of these issues is critical to recruitment, retention, and patient satisfaction. Managing expectations is also important. At this stage in the understanding of disease pathophysiology, treatments are not expected to cure ALS even if they are successful in slowing the disease or improving symptoms. It is critical that patients and families have a realistic understanding of what to expect in a trial.

Finally, clinical researchers can advocate with sponsors to offer open-label access for trial participants once the blinded phase of the trial is complete, assuming a positive result from early analysis. Independent of issues in trial design, actively engaging patients in the research process serves both the search for new treatments and the desires of patients to contribute to that effort. The importance of that active engagement extends beyond clinical trials. Enrolling in a data registry or contributing to a specimen bank are contributions every patient can make, and are contributions that may have as much importance in the ultimate development of a successful therapy as participation in a drug trial.

References

1 Chen Z, Turner MR: The internet for self-diagnosis and prognostication in ALS. Amyotroph Lateral Scler 2010;11: 565–567.
2 Landro: The informed patient.' Wall Street Journal, June 2007.
3 Wicks P, Massagli M, Frost J, et al: Sharing health data for better outcomes on PatientsLikeMe. J Med Internet Res 2010;12:e19.
4 NEALS: Fourth Annual Clinical Research Learning Institute in Clearwater Beach, FL. 2014. http://alsconsortium. org/news_CRLI_Clearwater_2014.php.
5 Gordon PH, Moore DH, Miller RG, et al: Efficacy of minocycline in patients with amyotrophic lateral sclerosis: a phase III randomized trial. Lancet Neurol 2007;6: 1045–1053.

Lucie I. Bruijn, PhD, MBA
ALS Association
1275 K Street, Suite 250
Washington, DC 20005 (USA)
E-Mail lucie@alsa-national.org

Beghi E, Logroscino G (eds): The Right Therapy for Neurological Disorders. From Randomized Trials to Clinical Practice.
Front Neurol Neurosci. Basel, Karger, 2016, vol 39, pp 154–162 (DOI: 10.1159/000445456)

General Overview, Conclusions, and Future Directions

Ettore Beghi[a] · Giancarlo Logroscino[b, c]

[a]Laboratory of Neurological Disorders, IRCCS-Mario Negri Institute for Pharmacological Research, Milan, [b]Department of Basic Medical Sciences, Neuroscience and Sense Organs, University of Bari 'Aldo Moro', Bari, and [c]Unit of Neurodegenerative Diseases, Department of Clinical Research in Neurology, University of Bari 'Aldo Moro', 'Pia Fondazione Cardinale G. Panico', Tricase, Italy

Abstract

Background: The traditional design of the randomized clinical trial (RCT) is challenged by the peculiarities of the genotype and phenotype of neurological disorders. **Summary:** RCTs are intended to verify the net effect of an investigational treatment on the outcome of a disease. This implies the inclusion of strictly homogeneous sample of patients that represent only in part the full disease spectrum. For this reason, pragmatic trials on representative samples of the general population are welcome. In neurodegenerative disorders, RCTs are generally performed in symptomatic individuals, when the pathologic process is already in course. Although genetic, biological and structural markers are the ideal instruments to detect the disease at a preclinical stage, the development of biomarkers is still in its infancy and even identified markers require in most of cases validation. Given the limited duration of an RCT, prospective studies with prolonged follow-up in well-defined inception cohorts are needed to assess the effectiveness of the treatment in all affected individuals seen in everyday practice. RCT are conducted mainly in Caucasians excluding other ethnicities. The difference of brain biology between men and women are still underestimated in RCTs. Patients, treating physicians, pharmaceutical companies, and regulatory authorities have differing needs, which may have important implications in planning and conducting RCTs. New therapeutic approaches are represented by personalized and precision medicine. Although largely investigational, these approaches may challenge the traditional RCT design. **Key Messages:** All those interested in the development of new treatments and treatment strategies for neurological disorders should be involved when planning an RCT and ad-hoc designs should be developed to address the peculiarities of neurological disorders. Differences in age, sex and ethnicity should have a primary role in the design of an RCT. The traditional structure of the RCT should be also revised taking into account the new perspectives of personalized and precision medicine.

© 2016 S. Karger AG, Basel

The randomized clinical trial (RCT) remains the mainstay to confirm the efficacy, safety, and tolerability of any new treatment in medicine. The treatment of neurological disorders is no exception. The basic structure of the RCT is illustrated in the chapter by Beghi [this vol., pp. 1–7]. The RCT is structured to verify in a limited period of time whether or not a given treatment is effective, ineffective, and/or noxious in a well-defined sample of patients affected by a given clinical condition, after controlling for the most relevant sources of bias (internal validity). However, these prerequisites are in conflict with a number of factors that characterize the onset and course of several neurological conditions [Beghi et al., this vol., pp. 8–23]. These include the age, sex, and ethnicity of the affected individuals; timing of the diagnosis, presence of biomarkers and concurrent clinical conditions, course and complications, and (not least) the overall severity of the disease. Several neurological conditions are characterized by an initial subclinical phase followed by an overt clinical phase, which may vary across patients, and a course that follows differing patterns. These factors have differing implications for the structure of the RCT and the related results.

Diagnosis

The main issues related to the diagnosis include the diagnostic criteria, presence of biomarkers, time lapse between the pathologic and the clinical onset, and variability of the clinical presentation [Logroscino et al., this vol., pp. 24–36]. As most neurological conditions differ with reference to these factors, each of them is likely to influence to a differing extent the response to a given treatment. Diagnostic criteria used in RCTs are mostly represented by lists of symptoms and signs that, according to the type and number, qualify a case as definite, probable, or possible. Some of these symptoms and signs may be absent in the early phase of the disease, thus preventing the inclusion of a case in the trial and favoring the inclusion of patients with a clinical condition other than the one targeted by the treatment in question. In addition, the capability to make a correct diagnosis in the early phase of a disease is reflected by the background and experience of the investigator along with his/her familiarity with the diagnostic criteria selected for the inclusion in the trial. Therefore, the recruit-

ing center may be an important source of bias unless the local investigators are properly trained. The issue is even more complicated when diagnostic biomarkers are used, as – except for neuroimaging (see below) – positive and negative predictive values are suboptimal in several cases.

Neurodegenerative disorders are a typical example in which early treatment is mandatory to contrast the pathological process at a time in which the nervous system is, at least in part, preserved. However, early treatment implies the recruitment of patients not presenting the diagnosis of interest and exclusion from the trial of patients not yet fully satisfying the diagnostic criteria. In this context, one must decide to what extent false-positive diagnoses should be accepted. This issue, which can be satisfactorily addressed by the randomization process, has ethical implications and may have a relevant effect on the occurrence of the end points chosen to test treatment efficacy.

Age, Sex, and Ethnicity

The worldwide population is aging and, for this reason, several chronic neurological conditions are going to increase. Paradoxically, patients enrolled in RCTs are rarely represented by elderly subjects. The obstacles to the enrolment of aged individuals in RCTs are clearly outlined in the chapter by Novy and Sander [this vol., pp. 71–80]. However, as with children, the exclusion of the elderly from therapeutic trials prevents them from experiencing benefits and harms of the investigational products, which are left to the use in clinical practice, thus exposing these individuals to the risks of treatment without knowing if that same treatment does help them.

Although RCTs rarely show different results in men and women, theoretically the effects of a treatment may differ in the two sexes. Men and women have a different life expectancy, differing comorbidities, and different exposure to several risk factors. These differences are even more evident when comparing individuals of different ethnic origin. Unfortunately, the role of ethnicity on the effects of treatments has been poorly investigated in the past and, as with age, non-Caucasian people may be unduly exposed to the effects of treatments without being included in RCTs.

Biomarkers

An increasing number of biomarkers has been investigated in RCTs on neurological disorders. Biomarkers have been used not only to identify affected individuals at a preclinical stage, but also to verify the effects of treatments on the presumed mechanisms of a disease. The chapter by Parnetti et al. [this vol., pp. 117–123] outlines the present knowledge on cerebrospinal fluid (CSF) biomarkers as signatures for Alzheimer's disease (AD) and Parkinson's disease (PD), and for target engagement in RCTs. In AD, three CSF biomarkers ($A\beta_{42}$, total tau, and phosphorylated tau) are used to support the diagnosis in the prodromal stages of the disease and to predict the progression to dementia in patients with mild cognitive impairment (core AD biomarkers). The investigation of other potentially useful markers (of neural injury, inflammation, or synaptic loss) is in progress, but their predictive value is still unknown. α-Synuclein is the most intensively investigated biomarker in PD. Mutations in the α-synuclein gene have been associated with PD, suggesting a central role of this protein in the disease process. Other biomarkers are also being studied. These include GBA1 (the gene encoding for the lysosomal enzyme glucocerebrosidase) and markers of oxidative stress, inflammation, and energy failure.

Current CSF biomarkers of AD are useful in RCTs to enrich patient samples and demonstrate target engagement. However, the association between the effects of drugs on these biomarkers and clinical outcomes has not been confirmed. In PD, the development of biomarkers is still in progress, but standardization of procedures and valid cutoffs are far from being defined. Novel biomarkers are needed in both clinical conditions.

In contrast to CSF, imaging represents a more robust source of biomarkers in the assessment of neurodegenerative diseases. Magnetic resonance imaging (MRI) has been reported in the chapter by Whitwell [this vol., pp. 101–108] as a fundamental tool not only to exclude other clinical conditions, but also as a marker of disease progression. MRI has advantages over clinical scales in being objective and not affected by floor and ceiling effects. For different neurodegenerative disorders, including AD, dementia with Lewy bodies, frontotemporal dementia, progressive supranuclear palsy, and PD associated with mild cognitive impairment or dementia, rates of temporal lobe atrophy, selective subcortical brain atrophy and/or posterior cerebral atrophy are indexes of disease progression in the prodromal, preclinical and early clinical phases. Using MRI as a biomarker, the required sample size is generally smaller than with clinical indicators of disease progression. However, MRI measures suffer from limitations such as dropouts, change over normal aging, and use of multisite data. Other MRI modalities are a source of future biomarkers. These include diffusion tensor imaging, task-free functional MRI, and arterial spin labeling. These modalities require validation.

As indicated in the chapter by Singhal and Stern [this vol., pp. 109–116], positron emission tomography (PET) and single-photon emission computed tomography (SPECT) precede conventional imaging technique in the detection of abnormalities because functional and molecular changes often precede structural changes. In light of their capabilities, these techniques are diagnostic, prognostic, and markers of disease activity as well as drug kinetics and effects.

In PD, [^{123}I]β-CIT is a SPECT tracer binding to presynaptic dopamine transporters with specific uptake in normal putamen and caudate.

[^{18}F]Fluorodopa is a PET tracer with presynaptic uptake in the basal ganglia reflecting the enzymatic activity of DOPA decarboxylase in dopaminergic terminals. Both tracers are decreased in PD. Posterior putamen is involved first, followed by the other basal ganglia as disease progresses. However, a decrease in radiotracer binding is observed with levodopa, revealing opposite results with reference to the effects of levodopa on PD. Then a correlation between the UPDRS scores and the radioligands is inconsistent. In addition, [^{18}F]fluorodopa may underestimate and [^{123}I] β-CIT may overestimate neuronal loss in the early stages of the disease and [^{123}I]β-CIT binding declines with age.

In AD, several [^{11}C]- and [^{18}F]-labeled radiopharmaceuticals have been developed. However, in RCTs a discrepancy was found between PET biomarker changes and clinical response. A possible explanation is that these techniques measure amyloid plaque burden, while in the preclinical course of AD the neurotoxic mechanisms are represented by the fibrillary forms of β-amyloid. Radioligands targeting the tau protein are in development.

In patients with internal carotid stenosis, increased oxygen extraction fraction, determined on [$^{0-15}$]H$_2$O-PET and [$^{0-15}$]O$_2$-PET, was used to select individuals who could benefit from the external carotid-internal carotid anastomosis in an RCT. However, due to the premature termination of the trial for a significantly increased rate of ipsilateral stroke, the role of this biomarker could not be definitely assessed.

In light of the present findings, for various reasons PET and SPECT techniques cannot yet be used as surrogate end points in RCTs. The parameters to be measured should reflect key mechanisms of the diseases to be targeted by the experimental drugs. Then the techniques still require standardization, they should be adapted to adjust for physiological changes occurring over time, and the expected changes should occur in the time frame of the trial.

Pharmacogenetics

In the last decades, genetics has given an important contribution to the understanding of the mechanisms involved in neurodegenerative diseases. As indicated in the chapter by Tortelli et al. [this vol., pp. 124–135], genetic factors may be implicated as the cause of the disease, may be involved with other factors in the pathophysiology, or may interact with treatments. The direct or indirect implication of genetic factors may have a profound influence on the clinical manifestations and the course of a disease and, for this reason, they must be considered when planning an RCT. In addition, genetic markers may be useful to identify presymptomatic carriers and patients at higher risk of disease or in the early phase of a disease, who represent the ideal target for early treatment. The mutation of the genes associated with a dominant form of early-onset AD (like the PSEN-1 E280A) lead to early amyloid plaque deposition followed by progressive cognitive decline several decades before the typical onset of the disease. Carriers of these mutated genes are now included in RCTs assessing the role of different antiamyloid monoclonal antibodies.

Apolipoprotein E (APOE) is the strongest phenotypic modifier in late-onset AD and, at present, the only genetic marker affecting drug response. APOE ε4 carriers treated with bapineuzumab present a decreased rate of accumulation of cortical amyloid. In addition, the gene TOMM40, in linkage disequilibrium with the APOE ε4 allele, is associated with an earlier age at onset of AD. Using this genetic marker, an ongoing RCT is testing the effect of pioglitazone in delaying the onset of mild cognitive impairment.

A mutation of the gene C90rf72 is the most frequent genetic abnormality in familial and sporadic forms of frontotemporal dementia and amyotrophic lateral sclerosis (ALS). However, no genetic biomarkers have been identified for frontotemporal dementia. Decreased plasma levels of

progranulin have been identified in GRN mutation carriers suggesting a loss of progranulin
function and the potential benefits of drugs increasing progranulin concentration, like chloroquine, nimodipine, and vorinostat.

The contribution of genetics for RCTs in patients with ALS is in its infancy. However, emerging technologies in antisense oligonucleotides
and RNA silencing may lead to the development
of treatments targeting specific genes in familial
ALS.

In PD, the response to L-DOPA and dopamine
agonists is largely determined by the genetic
background of the affected individuals. However,
for several reasons it has been impossible to identify dopamine-related polymorphisms affecting
treatment response. In Huntington's disease, despite the established genetic origin, the strategies
aimed at contrasting the deleterious effects of
mutant huntingtin protein are still under investigation.

Genetic factors play a relevant role in drug metabolism and, for this reason, the genetic background must be investigated to explain interindividual differences in drug response. The cytochrome P450 superfamily is the most important
class of genetic factors influencing treatment response. Several drugs used for the treatment of
PD activate or inhibit cytochrome P450 enzyme
functions, with important effects on their efficacy
and tolerability. For any investigational compound, drug metabolism and the possible interactions with the cytochrome P450 enzymes should
be investigated for a correct interpretation of the
effects of treatment.

Age and Comorbidity

Age and comorbidity are constantly taken into
account when planning an RCT. Older age and
presence of comorbidities are exclusion criteria in
most RCTs. However, in an aging population, elderly individuals are going to represent the largest
fraction of individuals affected by chronic neurological conditions. As a result, ageing is associated
with an increasing number of concurrent diseases. For these reasons, RCTs should consider the
inclusion of these patients. As clearly indicated in
the chapter by Novy and Sander [this vol., pp. 71–
80], psychiatric and somatic comorbidities are a
frequent occurrence in patients with neurological
disorders. Comorbidities may be the underlying
cause, another manifestation of the underlying
process, the consequence of the disease, or the
consequence of its treatment. With the presence
of comorbidities, the outcome of the disease may
be aggravated, with increased disability and premature mortality. Comorbidities themselves may
require treatments potentially interfering with
the investigational drug.

The inclusion of elderly individuals and patients with comorbidities in RCTs represents a serious complication of the study design. However,
even in trials dealing with very homogeneous
study samples, the influence of comorbidities
cannot be completely excluded. Perhaps RCTs focusing on elderly patients should be undertaken
and become part of the investigational therapeutic plan.

Disease Course, Outcome Measures, and
Prognostic Predictors

Along with age and comorbidities, other pheno-
typical aspects must be considered in the disease
course to explain (and predict) the outcome in order to assess the net effects of an investigational
treatment. In this book, two clinical conditions,
multiple sclerosis (MS) and epilepsy, are used as
examples to illustrate the heterogeneity of the
opening manifestations, the clinical course and
the outcome. As outlined in the chapter by Martinelli Boneschi and Comi [this vol., pp. 93–100],
MS is characterized by two main courses: bout-
onset MS (present in about 85% of cases) and progressive-onset MS (15% of cases). Bout-onset MS

presents with a relapsing-remitting course followed by secondary progression of the disease in the majority of cases. All available disease-modifying treatments have clear effects on the relapses, but at present none of them has been found to have a significant impact on the progressive phase. A possible explanation of the failure of the available compounds on the progression of the disease is the limited time lapse. Even when a prolonged follow-up of patients enrolled in the original trial is considered, the longitudinal observation may be too short for detecting changes in the conventional disability measures. This might be the case for the compounds not tested in patients with progressive-onset MS. The chapter's authors stress the importance of long-term observational studies and divide them in two major categories: concurrent cohort studies and historical cohort studies. The potential for bias (greater in historical than in concurrent cohort studies) is discussed. However, even with these limitations, observational studies are a valuable complement to the RCTs. These studies should include homogeneous inception cohorts, well-defined diagnostic criteria, use of matched controls, blind assessors of treatment efficacy and safety, use of hard end points, and predefined check-lists of common adverse events.

The limitations of the current RCTs are also emphasized in the field of epilepsy, a chronic clinical condition characterized by a pleomorphic course and a high rate of spontaneous remission [Schmidt, this vol., pp. 81–92]. Using data from a population-based study of patients with epilepsy started in infancy or childhood, the chapter's author identified patients with variable disease severity and differing prognostic patterns that must be considered when assessing treatment efficacy. Drugs used for the treatment of epilepsy are symptomatic compounds with virtually no effect of the course of the disease. The present structure of RCTs of antiepileptic drugs is contentious and suggestions have been made on how to improve the existing models by introducing antiepilepto-genic drugs, confronting the experimental drug with another active principle, and using seizure freedom as a major outcome measure. Biomarkers (as yet unavailable) that can predict high morbidity risk and poor seizure outcome must also be found. Outcomes may be represented by composite end-points, like in stroke research [Pistoia et al., this vol., pp. 60–70]. However, outcome measures vary across RCTs making it difficult to compare results.

Randomized Trials in Developing Countries

Patients living in developing countries represent a growing target population for RCTs. An extensive systematic review of published RCTs done in developing countries is presented in the chapter by Marin et al. [this vol., pp. 136–146]. The clinical conditions tested in the trials included infectious diseases, epilepsy and other paroxysmal disorders, and neurodegenerative diseases. Asia, Africa, and Latin America were, in decreasing order, the sites where the trials are organized and conducted. Only phase IIb and III trials were performed. The quality of the experiments was variable and generally suboptimal, with defects mostly involving randomization procedure, blinding, intent-to-treat analysis, and sample size calculation. The results of the review highlight the need to develop highly equipped structures dedicated to the early investigation of drugs in humans (to undertake phase I and IIa trials). The local investigators should also be trained to improve the methodological quality of study protocols, data management, statistical analysis, and scientific reports.

Statistical Methods and Significance

Given the heterogeneity of the disease, there was a discussion on the role of stratified medicine in defining population subgroups according to differences in prognosis and treatment response.

The difference can rely on clinical and demographical characteristics, genetic background, and biomarkers. However, a clear distinction is necessary to understand whether such aspects represent prognostic factors and/or treatment effects modifiers (i.e. variables affecting the response to treatment). Therefore, risk stratification ('prognostic trees') and covariate-treatment interaction detection are assessable ('interaction or predictive trees') [Copetti et al., this vol., pp. 50–59]. In this case, the partitioning algorithm recursively searches within the candidate covariates for the two subgroups in which the heterogeneity in treatment effect is maximized. Once a prognostic tree is built on the control arm, it can be used in the whole sample to understand whether or not treatment effect modifiers are present. Subgroups of patients can be identified in the early phase of a trial, and eventually tested in adaptive designs.

The most common application of tree-growing algorithms is their retrospective use to analyze RCTs who failed to prove overall efficacy and where preplanned subgroup analyses might as well have missed the chance to detect any statistically significant treatment effect. A tree-structure is the natural framework to understand and derive an evidence-based treatment algorithm, especially when dealing with more than one treatment. Further advances correspond to extend tree-growing techniques to real life data sources. By accounting for the clustered nature of some designs (e.g. multicenter observational studies), we would be able to address the role of the prescribers and whether or how they influence an evidence-based treatment algorithm derived in an RCT framework.

The role of statistics is not just limited to modeling and prediction, but also implies inference on the basis of data collection, processing, and analysis. The issue is discussed in the chapter by Bennett [this vol., pp. 37–49]. Statistical inference implies drawing conclusions about a population based on a sample of that population. Hypothesis testing, significance levels, and precision of the estimates are the key elements of the statistical reasoning to be considered when assessing the design and results of an RCT. Of note, statistical significance measures how likely it is that the observed differences in outcome between the treatment and control groups are real and not chance findings. Clinical significance measures how large the differences in effect size must be in clinical practice. Several attempts have been made to combine statistical and clinical significance. One suggested method is the minimal clinical important difference of the intervention to a point estimate and its confidence interval, according to which clinical importance can be stratified as 'definite', 'probable', 'possible', and 'definitely not'. A metric named the 'fragility index' has also been created to identify the number of events in an RCT required to change statistically significant results to nonsignificant results. In addition, Bayesian techniques have been proposed for situations in which conventional statistical approaches may be difficult or misleading. Graphical approaches combining statistical and clinical significance (relative risks, absolute risk reduction, number needed to treat) are also briefly discussed.

Patients' and Investigators' Expectations and Needs

Patients' involvement in the design, outcomes, and risk/benefit assessment is increasingly being recognized. Taking ALS for example, the chapter by Bruijn and Kolb [this vol., pp. 147–153] discusses the perspectives of people living with the disease and their perceptions of RCTs. The authors describe different organizations and programs available that impart education and encourage patient involvement. They envisage stronger partnerships between patients, clinicians, government, nonprofit organizations, and regulatory agencies to improve treatment development.

Conclusions and Future Directions

RCTs provide evidence on whether drugs or other therapeutic interventions result in improved outcomes in samples of patients obtained to minimize random error and control bias. However, the study design, which is intended to verify the net effect of treatment on the outcome of the disease, is in conflict with the heterogeneity of the clinical manifestations and course of most neurological disorders. For this reason, pragmatic trials including more representative samples of affected individuals in the general population are welcome. In such studies, heterogeneity could be controlled by including prognostic trees and interaction and predictive trees in the statistical analysis plan.

Most RCTs are performed in symptomatic individuals when the progression of the disease hampers the therapeutic potential of drugs potentially acting on the underlying pathophysiological mechanisms. Genetic, biological, and structural markers represent ideal instruments to identify disease onset and course at a preclinical stage. However, the development of biomarkers is still in its infancy and even the markers so far identified require proper validation before being used in RCTs.

Another important limitation of an RCT is represented by the limited duration of the trial. Cohort studies with prolonged follow-up can be valuable complementary studies to the RCTs. Although the limitations of cohort studies are well-known, the use of well-defined inception cohorts, a prospective design, objective end points, and robust statistical methods are a good compromise to improve the external validity of the results.

Patients, treating physicians, pharmaceutical companies, and regulatory authorities have differing needs and expectations. These needs and expectations can be hardly reconciled and may differ according to the clinical condition. However, all these actors should be involved when planning and conducting an RCT and ad hoc designs should be developed to address the variable genotypic and phenotypic aspects of neurological conditions.

The Randomized Clinical Trial in the Era of Personalized and Precision Medicine

Personalized medicine refers to an approach of clinical work where a treatment or a procedure is not chosen based on the 'average patient belonging to a group', but on the specific characteristics of that individual patient. Precision medicine, a strategy that takes into account prevention and treatment of individual variability, has been part of a systematic effort launched by President Obama in the US [1]. Both personalized and precision medicine are indicating a new general approach to medicine in clinical practice and in biomedical research. This is the consequence of a change in knowledge of the last few years due to genome-wide association studies, metabolomics, epigenomics, and epidemiology based on new international databases. There is still an important gap between these paths of possible future perspectives and what we really do. In reality we use some characteristics of the patient (especially genetic profile) to implement a better characterization of the individual patient as part of a large or small group sharing the same characteristics. If we have more than a single feature, our ability to describe the individual patient improves.

This approach will be extraordinarily important in the world of RCTs. However, even in presence of this new approach, we have to underline that the road from the laboratory to the RCT in humans is in most cases characterized by too many failures in neurology, especially in the area of neurodegenerative diseases. This is not the case in other areas of medicine. Recent advancements in the knowledge of biomarkers has in fact deeply changed the scenario of RCTs in oncology.

The traditional structure of four-phase RCTs with a placebo arm has been challenged. The RCT involves a large numbers of patients and neither the patient nor the clinician has any clue about the drug the randomized subject is taking. Large numbers of people, a lot of time, and millions of dollars are invested in these enormous projects for testing new drugs. Many researchers suggest a more flexible approach with a preliminary phase to get a quick possible answer [2].

The critical point is of course to find effective biomarkers of therapeutic response. In oncology there has been the case of critonizib in lymphoma and ALK/ELM4. In infectious diseases a very advanced scenario has been developed in hepatitis C to identify responders to traditional treatment [2]. To our knowledge there is no similar case in neurology.

Genome-wide association studies have not been very rewarding in terms of identification of biomarkers for therapeutic response in neurological diseases. Most biomarkers are based on a continuous scale and not on a binary scale (yes or no) that would be optimal to give a direct answer in the clinical decision process.

Based on the principle of personalized medicine, conventional phase III trials are largely inefficient. A very selected group of people is part of the trial, but the data on important characteristics of subjects are often missing (genetics and several lifestyle factors). After approval, this is one of several reasons to start a new RCT in a more selected group of subjects. Another consequence of the structure of the traditional RCT is that the number needed to treat is generally extraordinarily high [3]. For statins, this number is high as 10 and for Copaxone in MS it is 16. There is a future prospective for n of 1 trials where the same approach of clinical medicine will be tried with only 1 person experiencing the tested treatment.

These changes of perspective in RCTs have been applied mostly in other fields. To have similar progress in neurology, we need to keep aiming at the anticipation of the diagnosis, the development of valid biomarkers, and eventually at a new classification, especially of common diseases, as is already happening with AD. However, we think that the path to getting the neurological patients on the right drug with the right dose at the right time [4] is still quite long and difficult.

References

1 Collins FS, Varmus H: A new initiative on precision medicine. N Engl J Med 2015;372:793–795.

2 Vaidyanathan G: Redefining clinical trials: the age of personalized medicine. Cell 2012;148:1079–1080.

3 Schork NJ: Personalized medicine: time for one-person trials. Nature 2015;520: 609–611.

4 Hamburg MA, Collins FS: The path to personalized medicine. N Engl J Med 2010;363:301–304.

Ettore Beghi, MD
Laboratory of Neurological Disorders, IRCCS-Mario Negri Institute for Pharmacological Research
Via Giuseppe La Masa 19
IT–20156 Milan (Italy)
E-Mail ettore.beghi@marionegri.it

Author Index

Subject Index